INTERSTITIAL CYSTITIS

DIET COOKBOOK FOR BEGINNERS

Simple, Soothing Recipes and Expert Guidance for Managing Bladder Pain and Enhancing Well-Being

Kingsley Klopp

Table of Contents

Dinner Recipes

Soups and Salad Recipes

Snacks & Sides Recipes

To show our appreciation for your purchase, we're delighted to offer you these special bonuses as a heartfelt thank you.

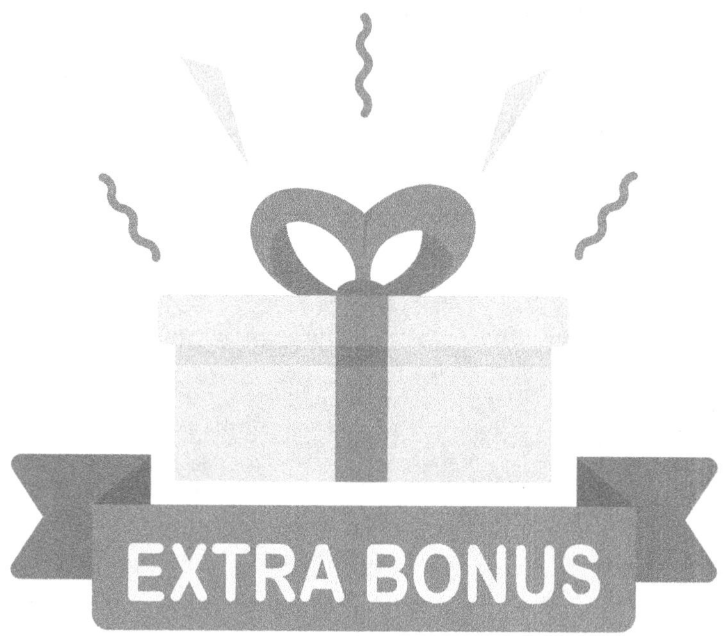

1. A Food Tracker Journal
2. Downloadable E-BOOK featuring full-color images of finished recipes

Important Note

Thank you for choosing the **Interstitial Cystitis Diet Cookbook for Beginners.** This cookbook is designed to help you navigate the challenges of living with interstitial cystitis through delicious, bladder-friendly recipes. As you embark on this culinary journey, please keep in mind that each person's experience with interstitial cystitis is unique, and dietary needs can vary significantly from one individual to another.

While the recipes in this cookbook are crafted to be gentle on the bladder and beneficial for those with interstitial cystitis, it's essential to listen to your body and adjust the ingredients to suit your specific needs. What works well for one person might not be suitable for another, and it's crucial to personalize your diet based on your own symptoms and triggers.

We strongly recommend consulting with your healthcare provider or a registered dietitian before making significant changes to your diet. They can provide personalized guidance and ensure that your dietary choices support your overall health and well-being. If you find yourself feeling uncertain or confused at any point, seeking professional advice is always a wise decision.

Please also note that the nutritional information provided for each recipe is approximate and may vary depending on the specific ingredients and brands you use. These figures are meant to serve as a general guide to help you make informed choices, but they should not be taken as exact measurements.

Furthermore, If our cookbook has brought joy to your kitchen and table, we'd be thrilled to hear about your experiences in an Amazon review. On the flip side, if you stumble upon any hiccups while exploring our recipes, don't hesitate to get in touch at **kloppkingsley@gmail.com.** We're here to support your cooking journey every step of the way.

Our goal is to empower you with the knowledge and tools to create meals that not only support your health but also bring joy and satisfaction to your table. We hope this cookbook becomes a valuable resource on your journey to managing interstitial cystitis with confidence and ease.
Wishing you good health and happy cooking,

Introduction.

Welcome to the **Interstitial Cystitis Diet Cookbook for Beginners.** If you've found yourself holding this book, you're likely on a challenging journey with interstitial cystitis (IC), a condition that can greatly impact your quality of life. Whether you're newly diagnosed or have been managing IC for some time, you know how crucial diet is in managing symptoms and improving your overall well-being. This cookbook is here to guide you through the complexities of eating for IC with compassion, support, and, most importantly, delicious recipes. Interstitial cystitis is more than just a medical condition; it's a daily struggle that affects your choices, your comfort, and your peace of mind. The pain, urgency, and frequency associated with IC can be overwhelming. Yet, amid these challenges, there is hope. Through thoughtful dietary adjustments, many people with IC have found significant relief, reducing symptoms and regaining control over their lives. This book is more than a collection of recipes. It's a beacon of hope and a practical guide designed to make your journey easier. Here, you'll find a treasure trove of bladder-friendly recipes that not only nourish your body but also bring joy to your taste buds. From soothing breakfasts and hearty lunches to comforting dinners and satisfying snacks, each recipe has been meticulously crafted to be both delicious and gentle on your bladder.

Our recipes are designed with the beginner in mind, ensuring that they are easy to follow, require accessible ingredients, and cater to a variety of tastes. But beyond the recipes, this cookbook offers valuable insights into understanding how different foods affect IC. You'll learn which ingredients to embrace and which to avoid, empowering you to make informed choices about your diet. Living with interstitial cystitis can sometimes feel isolating, but know that you are not alone. Many others have walked this path and have found strength and comfort in making positive dietary changes. As you explore these pages, you'll discover practical tips for navigating dining out, dealing with cravings, and staying motivated. Our goal is to make this transition as smooth and enjoyable as possible, helping you to reclaim your love for food without fear.

Set out on this culinary journey with an open heart and a hopeful spirit. Each meal is a step toward better health and a more vibrant life. The **Interstitial Cystitis Diet Cookbook for Beginner**s is here to support you every step of the way, offering comfort, inspiration, and a reminder that you can thrive, even with IC.

Thank you for allowing us to be part of your journey. Here's to your health, happiness, and delicious, bladder-friendly meals.

Warmest wishes,
Kingsley Klopp

Understanding Interstitial Cystitis and Diet

What is Interstitial Cystitis?

Interstitial cystitis, often abbreviated as IC and also known as painful bladder syndrome, is a condition that results in recurring discomfort or pain in the bladder and the surrounding pelvic region. Imagine feeling an urgent need to visit the bathroom numerous times throughout the day and night, or experiencing pain that ranges from mild to severe during bladder filling and relief upon emptying. That's the relentless cycle someone with interstitial cystitis might endure. This condition is somewhat enigmatic and frequently misunderstood, not only by those who suffer from it but also occasionally by the medical community. It's not caused by an infection, though it mimics urinary tract infections. Instead, it's a chronic, often debilitating condition that can significantly impact one's quality of life, affecting social interactions, work productivity, and mental health. One of the most profound aspects of IC is its emotional toll. Many sufferers report feeling frustrated and hopeless due to the persistent pain and the lack of a definitive cure. The constant search for a bathroom can lead to anxiety and stress, which only exacerbates the symptoms. It's a condition that can feel isolating, as the pain and urgency can make it challenging to engage in social activities or long events.

The exact cause of interstitial cystitis is still a subject of research, but several theories exist. Some suggest that it might be an autoimmune response, others consider a defect in the bladder tissue that allows irritating substances in the urine to penetrate its lining. There's also a belief that it could be related to an inflammatory condition of the pelvic nerves. This complexity means that diagnosing IC can be a lengthy process of eliminating other conditions like infections, bladder stones, or cancer.

Symptomatically, IC varies widely from person to person. The hallmark symptoms are persistent pain in the bladder and pelvic area, and a frequent, urgent need to urinate. Some may experience pain as their bladder fills, which somewhat diminishes after emptying it. Others report constant pain that varies in intensity throughout the day. The symptoms can fluctuate with periods of flares and remissions—times when the symptoms worsen and improve, respectively.

Women are more frequently diagnosed with IC than men, and symptoms can often be mistaken for other conditions such as chronic pelvic pain syndrome. In men, these symptoms can mimic chronic prostatitis or chronic pelvic pain syndrome. For both sexes, the emotional and physical toll can lead to significant lifestyle changes and adaptations to manage the symptoms.

Living with IC often means modifying many aspects of daily life, including diet. Many people with IC find that certain foods and beverages can trigger flares. Common culprits include caffeinated drinks, alcoholic beverages, tomatoes, spicy foods, and artificial sweeteners. However, triggers can vary widely, so individuals often need to keep detailed food diaries to identify what exacerbates their symptoms.

Treatment for IC is as individual as the condition itself. There is no one-size-fits-all solution, and what works for one person may not work for another. Treatments range from dietary modifications and physical therapy to medications and procedures that target the bladder's lining. Pain management is also a crucial component, addressing both the physical and emotional aspects of pain.

For those newly diagnosed with IC, it's important to seek support and education. Connecting with others who understand the nuances of living with IC can be invaluable. Support groups, whether online or in person, can provide a platform to share experiences, tips, and emotional support. Furthermore, working with healthcare providers who are knowledgeable about IC is critical. It often takes a team approach to effectively manage the symptoms and improve quality of life.

In summary, interstitial cystitis is more than just a medical condition; it's a complex, chronic issue that intertwines physical symptoms with emotional challenges. It demands a comprehensive management strategy that encompasses physical health, emotional resilience, and community support. For anyone grappling with this condition, remember, you are not alone, and with the right approach, you can manage the symptoms and lead a fulfilling life.

The Link Between Diet and IC

If you or someone you know is battling interstitial cystitis (IC), you've likely heard that what you eat can significantly affect your symptoms. This connection between diet and IC is not just about avoiding discomfort; it's about regaining control over one's life. It's about transforming the kitchen from a place of potential harm into a sanctuary of healing. Understanding the link between diet and IC starts with recognizing that the bladder is extraordinarily sensitive in those with the condition. Certain foods and beverages can irritate the bladder's lining, exacerbating the feelings of urgency, frequency, and pain that characterize IC. This is why diet modification often becomes a cornerstone of managing IC symptoms.

Now, let's talk about how this plays out in daily life. Imagine planning your day around proximity to restrooms, or feeling apprehensive about dining out for fear of a flare-up. The emotional toll of such constant vigilance is significant. It's not just about physical discomfort; it's about feeling anxious at the thought of eating the wrong thing and suffering the consequences. For many with IC, this means adopting an elimination diet to determine which foods trigger symptoms. Common irritants include tomatoes, citrus fruits, spicy foods, caffeine, and alcoholic beverages. But it's not the same for everyone—what might trigger a flare in one person could be perfectly fine for another. This individual variability adds a layer of complexity and frustration to managing the condition. It's a bit like being a detective in your own kitchen, trying to pinpoint what harms and what heals. The process can be isolating and overwhelming. Picture having to turn down your favorite meals or navigate social gatherings where the menu is out of your control. The fear of pain can lead to anxiety around food, which only compounds the stress of the condition.

However, it's not all about restrictions. Many find that embracing an IC-friendly diet opens up a new relationship with food. It becomes less about what you can't eat and more about what you can do to soothe your body. Foods like pears, blueberries, and carrots, as well as whole grains and lean proteins, can become staples that help maintain bladder health without causing discomfort.

Hydration is also a critical aspect. While it might seem counterintuitive to drink more when you feel like you're always looking for a bathroom, adequate water intake can help dilute urine and reduce irritation. It's about finding that balance where the water is enough to hydrate but not so much that it triggers more frequent trips to the bathroom.

The emotional journey of linking diet to symptom management is complex. There's the initial frustration and grief of altering one's diet, followed by the hopeful experimentation of adding and removing foods. And when a balance is found, there's a profound sense of relief and empowerment. Learning to manage IC through diet is not just about following a list of do's and don'ts; it's about reconnecting with your body, understanding its signals, and nurturing it in the most personal way.

Foods to Embrace and Avoid

When you're navigating life with interstitial cystitis (IC), your relationship with food transforms dramatically. What once may have been a source of pleasure can become a source of fear if you've experienced the painful consequences of a dietary misstep. But it's not just about fear; it's about forging a new, more mindful relationship with what you eat. This shift—recognizing which foods to embrace and which to avoid—can be a significant step toward managing your symptoms and reclaiming a sense of normalcy and joy in eating.

Foods to Avoid: Let's talk about the tough part first—the foods that are often better left uneaten for those with IC. The usual suspects here include:

1. **Citrus Fruits and Tomato-Based Products**: These are high in acid and can be very irritating to the bladder. That sharp, burning sensation during a flare can often be traced back to a lemonade or a tomato pasta sauce.
2. **Spicy Foods**: The heat that adds zest to your meals can unfortunately translate into painful heat in your bladder.
3. **Caffeine**: Found in coffee, tea, chocolate, and some sodas, caffeine is a major no-go for many with IC. It's a diuretic, which increases urine production and potentially the frequency of discomfort.
4. **Alcoholic Beverages**: Alcohol can irritate the bladder lining directly, worsening the symptoms.
5. **Artificial Sweeteners**: Whether it's in your diet soda or added to your coffee, artificial sweeteners like aspartame and saccharin have been known to cause flare-ups.

The thought of giving up these foods and drinks might make you feel a sense of loss. Social gatherings, holidays, or even a simple pleasure like a morning cup of coffee might now be tinged with anxiety or sadness over what you can't have. It's a valid feeling, reflecting the grief for a former way of life.

Foods to Embrace: But it's not all about avoidance; there's also a beautiful side to this new dietary journey—discovering foods that you can enjoy without fear. These include:

1. **Pears and Blueberries:** Among fruits, pears and blueberries are generally well-tolerated by those with IC. They can be a sweet, refreshing part of your diet without the fear of a flare.
2. **Root Vegetables:** Potatoes, carrots, and beets are nourishing and less likely to irritate your bladder. They can be roasted, mashed, or used in soups, providing both comfort and nutrition.
3. **Whole Grains:** Foods like bread, pasta, and cereals made from whole grains are usually safe for IC sufferers. They're also comforting and versatile.
4. **Mild Cheeses:** Unlike some aged cheeses, mild varieties such as mozzarella and ricotta are usually well tolerated and can add a delightful creaminess to your meals.
5. **Herbal Teas:** Herbal teas, particularly chamomile or peppermint, are soothing options that can help keep you hydrated without the risk associated with caffeinated beverages.

Embracing this new way of eating allows you to connect with your food in a deeper, more meaningful way. It becomes about nourishment, about healing, about taking control of your health. Yes, it requires adjustment and a significant amount of trial and error. Each person's triggers are unique, and the process of identifying yours can be fraught with frustration. However, there's also a sense of empowerment that comes with mastering your IC diet. You become more attuned to your body's needs and responses. Meals become opportunities to nourish and care for yourself, to prevent pain rather than inadvertently cause it. The joy of eating can be rediscovered through safe, soothing foods that help manage your symptoms and enhance your quality of life.

To those just starting this journey, be patient with yourself. It's a path of discovery, of learning what helps and what hurts. Embrace the challenge with an open heart, and let your diet be your ally in your fight against IC.

Breakfast Recipes

1. Pear Oatmeal

Ingredients:

- 1 cup rolled oats
- 2 cups water or oat milk
- 1 ripe pear, diced
- 1 tbsp honey or maple syrup
- 1/4 tsp cinnamon

Instructions:

1. In a small pot, bring the water or oat milk to a boil.
2. Add the oats and simmer for about 5 minutes, stirring occasionally.
3. Stir in the diced pear, honey (or maple syrup), and cinnamon.
4. Cook for another 5 minutes or until the oats are soft and creamy.

Nutrition Info Per Serving:

- Calories: 300
- Protein: 6g
- Carbohydrates: 60g
- Fat: 4g

Serves: 2
Cooking Time: 10 minutes

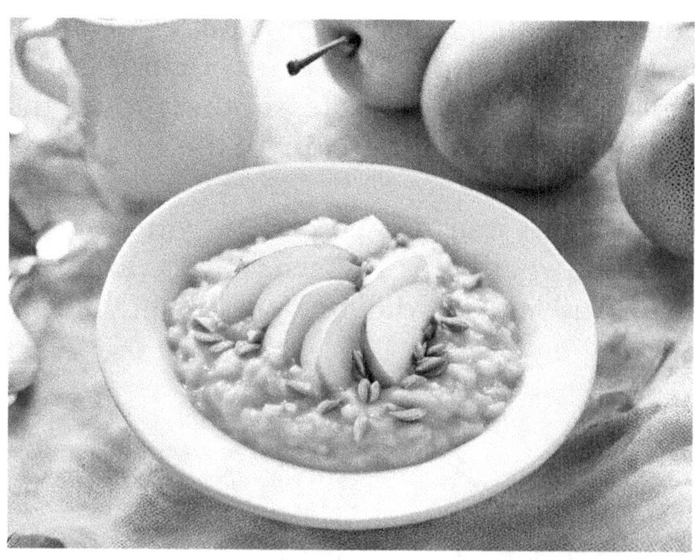

2. Blueberry Smoothie
Ingredients:
- 1 cup blueberries (fresh or frozen)
- 1 banana
- 1 cup unsweetened almond milk
- 1 tbsp flaxseeds

Instructions:
1. Combine all ingredients in a blender.
2. Blend on high until smooth.

Nutrition Info Per Serving:
- Calories: 180
- Protein: 3g
- Carbohydrates: 35g
- Fat: 4g

Serves: 2
Cooking Time: 5 minutes

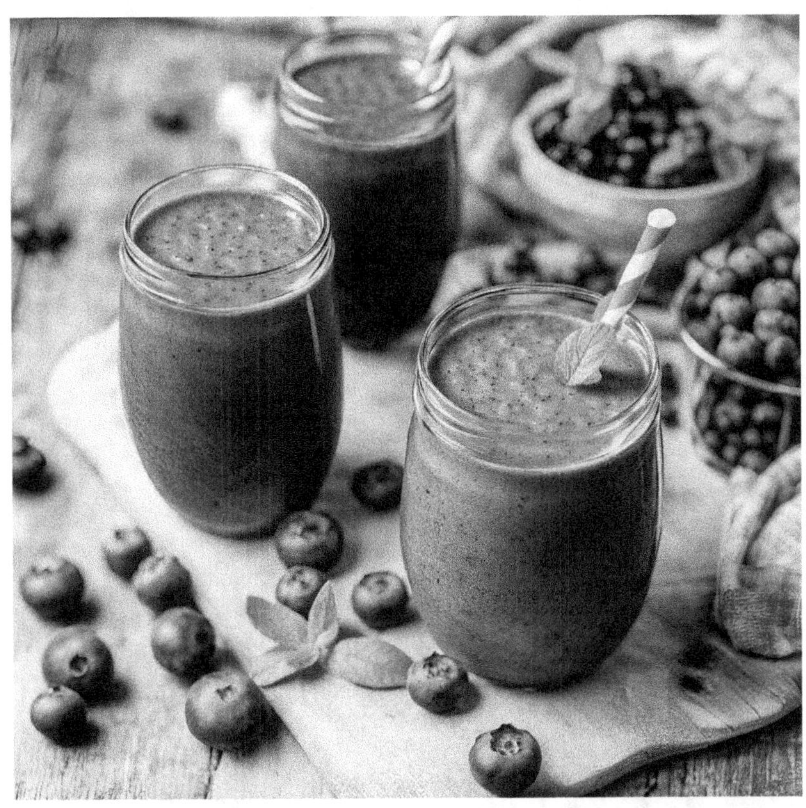

3. Banana Pancakes

Ingredients:

- 1 ripe banana, mashed
- 1 cup oat flour
- 1 tsp baking powder
- 1/2 cup almond milk
- 1 tbsp olive oil

Instructions:

1. In a bowl, mix the mashed banana, oat flour, and baking powder.
2. Gradually add almond milk to reach a batter consistency.
3. Heat olive oil in a pan and pour batter to form pancakes.
4. Cook until bubbles form on the surface, then flip and cook the other side.

Nutrition Info Per Serving:

- Calories: 250
- Protein: 5g
- Carbohydrates: 45g
- Fat: 7g

Serves: 2

Cooking Time: 10 minutes

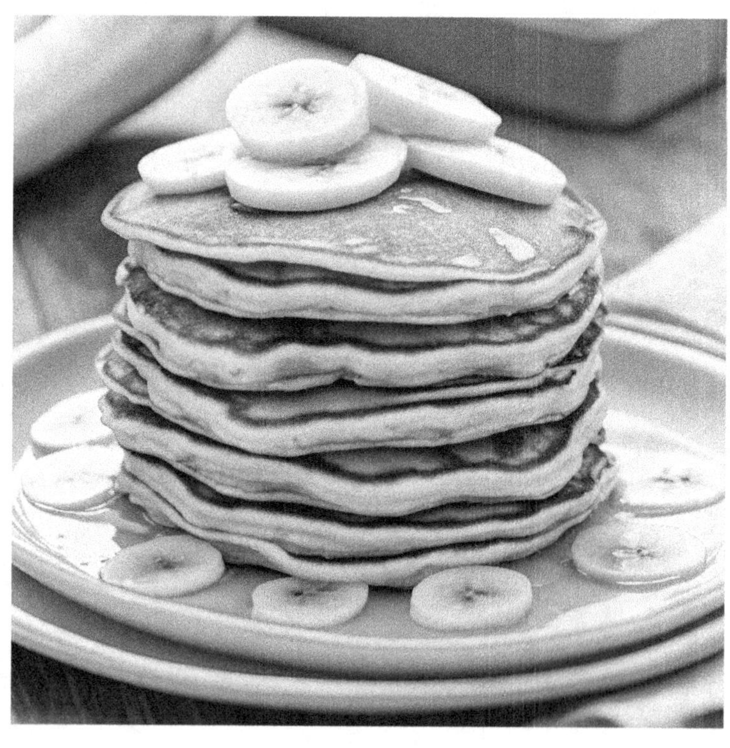

4. Apple Cinnamon Porridge
Ingredients:
- 1 cup rolled oats
- 2 cups water or almond milk
- 1 apple, peeled and chopped
- 1/4 tsp cinnamon
- 1 tbsp honey or maple syrup

Instructions:
1. In a pot, bring water or almond milk to a boil.
2. Add oats, chopped apple, and cinnamon.
3. Simmer until oats are tender and apples are soft, about 5-7 minutes.
4. Stir in honey or maple syrup before serving.

Nutrition Info Per Serving:
- Calories: 280
- Protein: 6g
- Carbohydrates: 55g
- Fat: 4g

Serves: 2
Cooking Time: 10 minutes

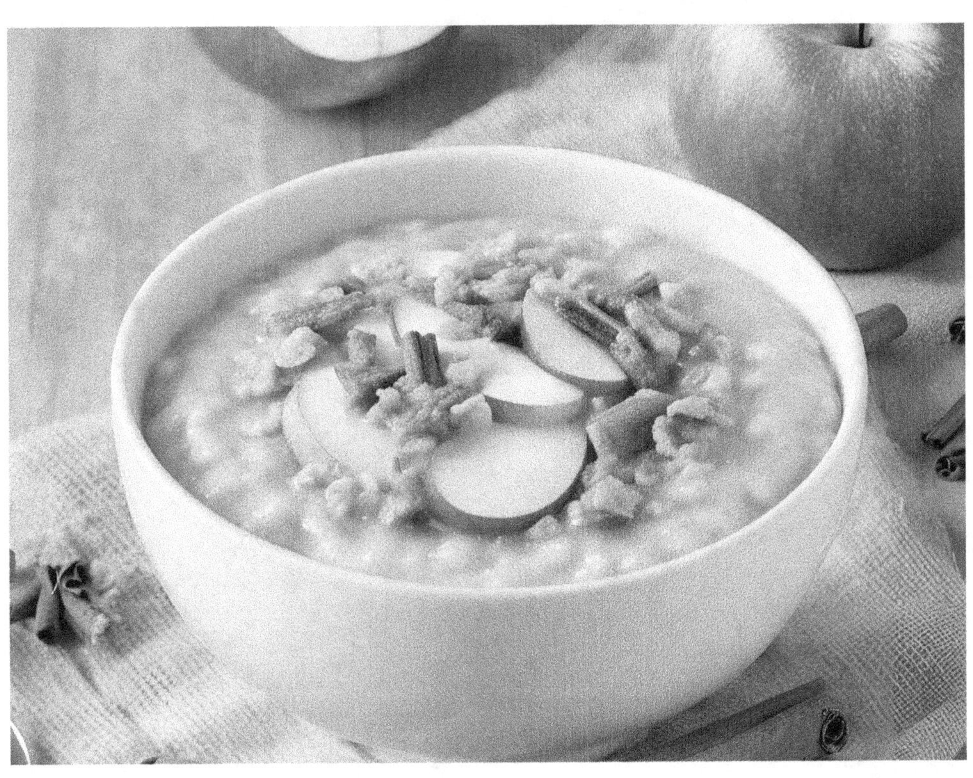

5. Rice Pudding

Ingredients:

- 1 cup cooked white rice
- 2 cups almond milk
- 2 tbsp honey or maple syrup
- 1/4 tsp cinnamon

Instructions:

1. In a pot, combine cooked rice with almond milk, honey, and cinnamon.
2. Cook over medium heat, stirring occasionally until thick and creamy.

Nutrition Info Per Serving:

- Calories: 200
- Protein: 4g
- Carbohydrates: 40g
- Fat: 2g

Serves: 2
Cooking Time: 20 minutes

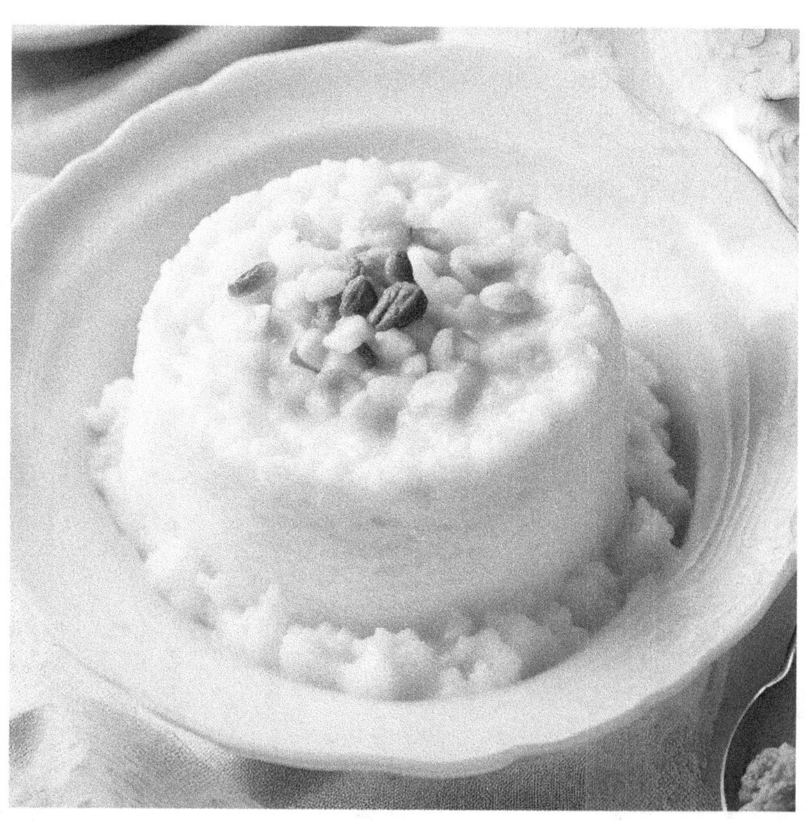

6. Pumpkin Oatmeal

Ingredients:

- 1 cup rolled oats
- 2 cups water or almond milk
- 1/2 cup pureed pumpkin (not pumpkin pie filling)
- 1 tbsp honey or maple syrup
- 1/4 tsp cinnamon

Instructions:

1. In a pot, bring the water or almond milk to a boil.
2. Add oats and pumpkin puree, and reduce to a simmer.
3. Stir in cinnamon and honey or maple syrup.
4. Cook until oats are tender, about 5 minutes.

Nutrition Info Per Serving:

- Calories: 300
- Protein: 6g
- Carbohydrates: 60g
- Fat: 4g

Serves: 2
Cooking Time: 10 minutes

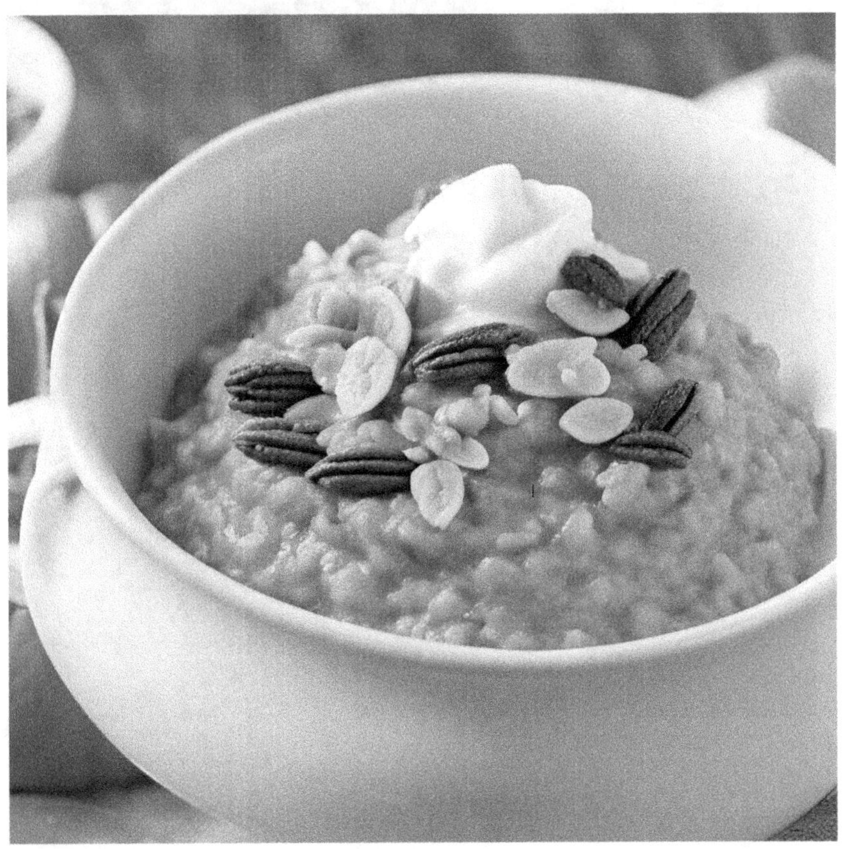

7. Avocado Rice Cakes

Ingredients:

- 2 rice cakes
- 1 ripe avocado, mashed
- 1 tbsp chia seeds
- 1 tbsp lemon juice

Instructions:

1. Spread mashed avocado evenly over rice cakes.
2. Sprinkle chia seeds and drizzle lemon juice on top.

Nutrition Info Per Serving:

- Calories: 240
- Protein: 4g
- Carbohydrates: 27g
- Fat: 14g

Serves: 2

Cooking Time: 5 minutes

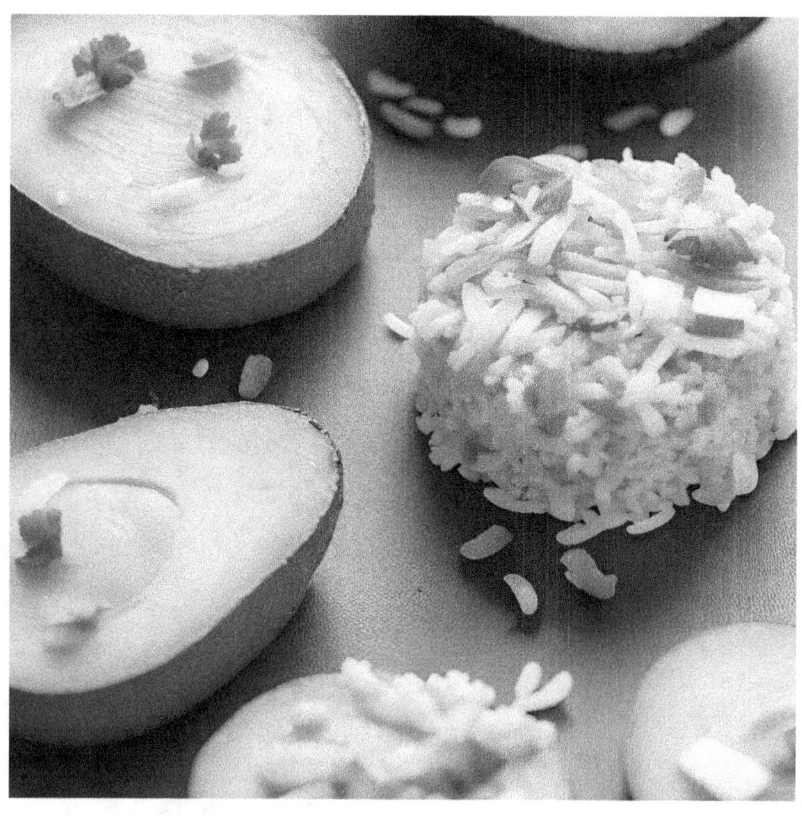

8. Sweet Potato Hash

Ingredients:

- 2 medium sweet potatoes, peeled and diced
- 1 tbsp olive oil
- 1/2 red bell pepper, diced
- 1/2 cup diced onion
- 1/4 tsp ground turmeric

Instructions:

1. Heat olive oil in a large skillet over medium heat.
2. Add sweet potatoes, bell pepper, and onion.
3. Cook, stirring occasionally, until the vegetables are tender and slightly browned, about 15 minutes.
4. Sprinkle turmeric and stir well for another minute.

Nutrition Info Per Serving:

- Calories: 220
- Protein: 3g
- Carbohydrates: 38g
- Fat: 7g

Serves: 4
Cooking Time: 15 minutes

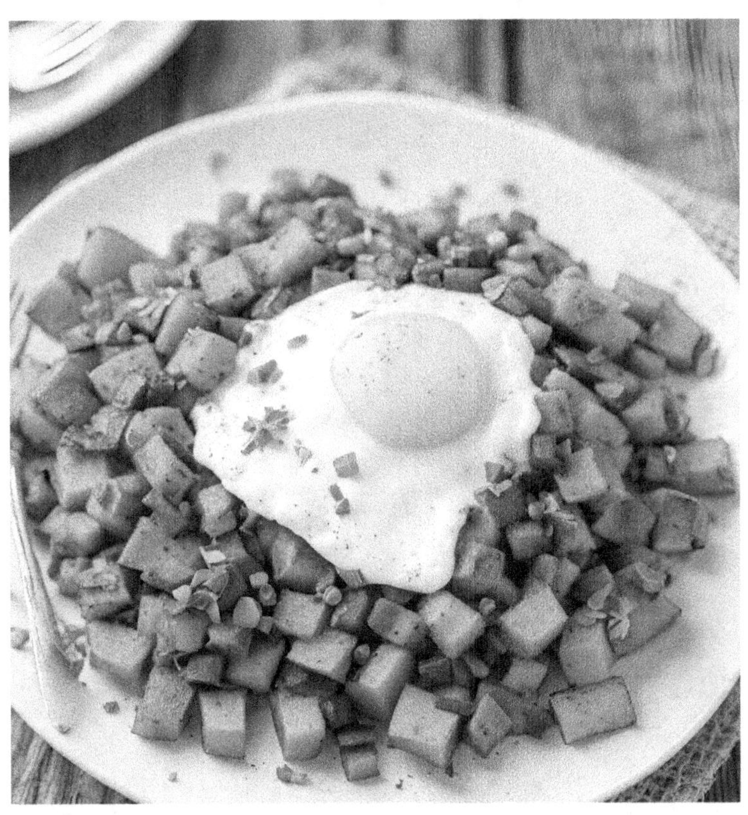

9. Zucchini Bread

Ingredients:

- 2 cups grated zucchini
- 1 cup oat flour
- 1/2 cup almond flour
- 1/4 cup olive oil
- 1/4 cup honey or maple syrup
- 1 tsp baking powder
- 1/4 tsp cinnamon

Instructions:

1. Preheat your oven to 350°F (175°C).
2. In a large bowl, combine grated zucchini, oat flour, almond flour, olive oil, honey, baking powder, and cinnamon.
3. Pour the batter into a greased loaf pan.
4. Bake for 50 minutes, or until a toothpick inserted into the center comes out clean.

Nutrition Info Per Serving:

- Calories: 200
- Protein: 4g
- Carbohydrates: 30g
- Fat: 8g

Serves: 8
Cooking Time: 50 minutes

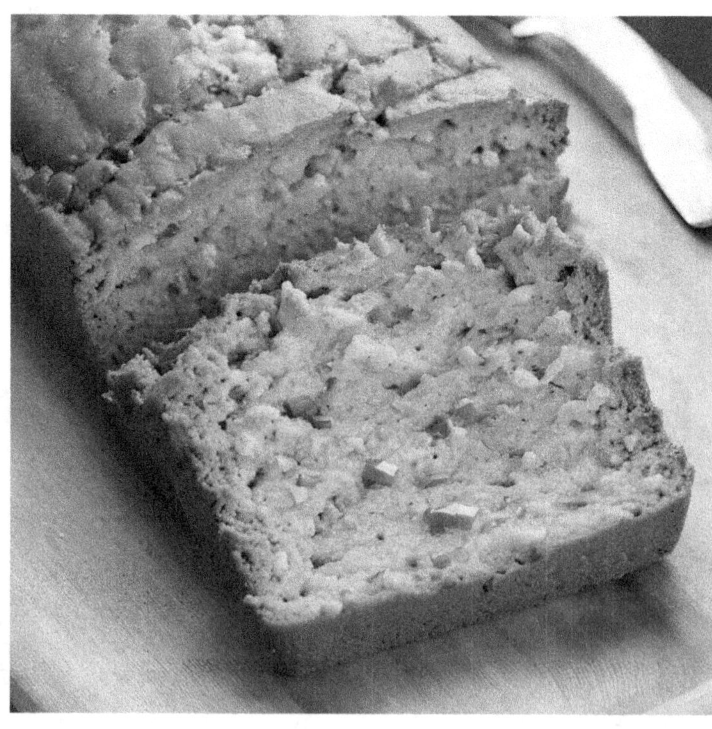

10. Oat Bran Porridge

Ingredients:

- 1 cup oat bran
- 2 cups water or almond milk
- 1 tbsp maple syrup
- 1/4 tsp ground cinnamon
- Fresh berries for topping (optional)

Instructions:

1. In a saucepan, bring the water or almond milk to a boil.
2. Add oat bran and reduce heat to a simmer.
3. Cook for about 5-7 minutes, stirring occasionally until the mixture thickens.
4. Stir in the maple syrup and cinnamon.
5. Serve hot, topped with fresh berries if desired.

Nutrition Info Per Serving:

- Calories: 150
- Protein: 6g
- Carbohydrates: 32g
- Fat: 2g

Serves: 2

Cooking Time: 10 minutes

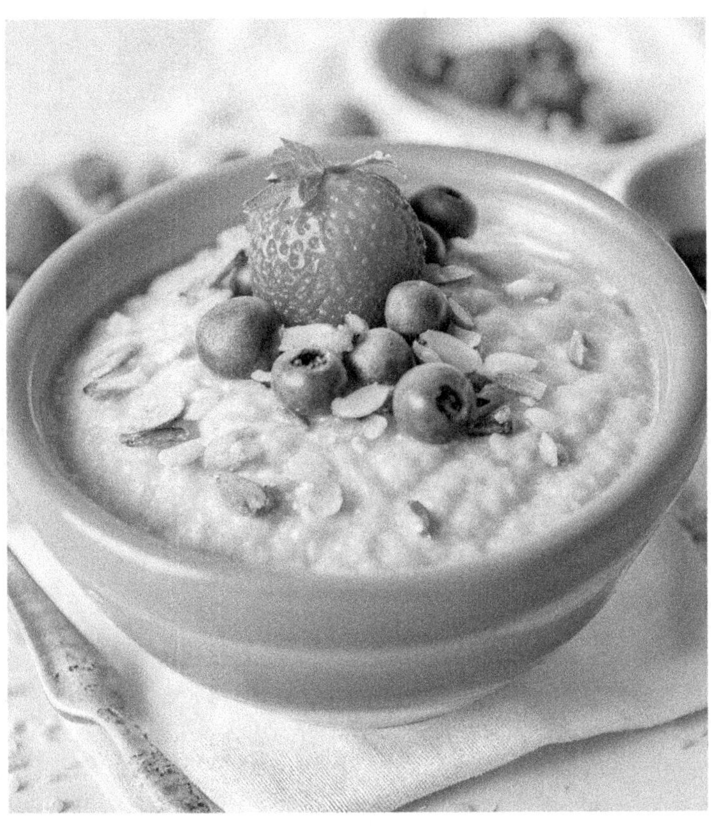

11. Millet Porridge

Ingredients:

- 1 cup millet, rinsed and drained
- 3 cups water
- 1/2 tsp ground cinnamon
- 1 tbsp honey or maple syrup
- 1/2 cup chopped nuts (such as almonds or walnuts)

Instructions:

1. In a medium saucepan, combine millet and water.
2. Bring to a boil, then reduce heat to low and simmer covered for 20 minutes.
3. Once cooked and water is absorbed, stir in cinnamon and honey or maple syrup.
4. Serve warm, sprinkled with chopped nuts.

Nutrition Info Per Serving:

- Calories: 215
- Protein: 6g
- Carbohydrates: 40g
- Fat: 5g

Serves: 4

Cooking Time: 25 minutes

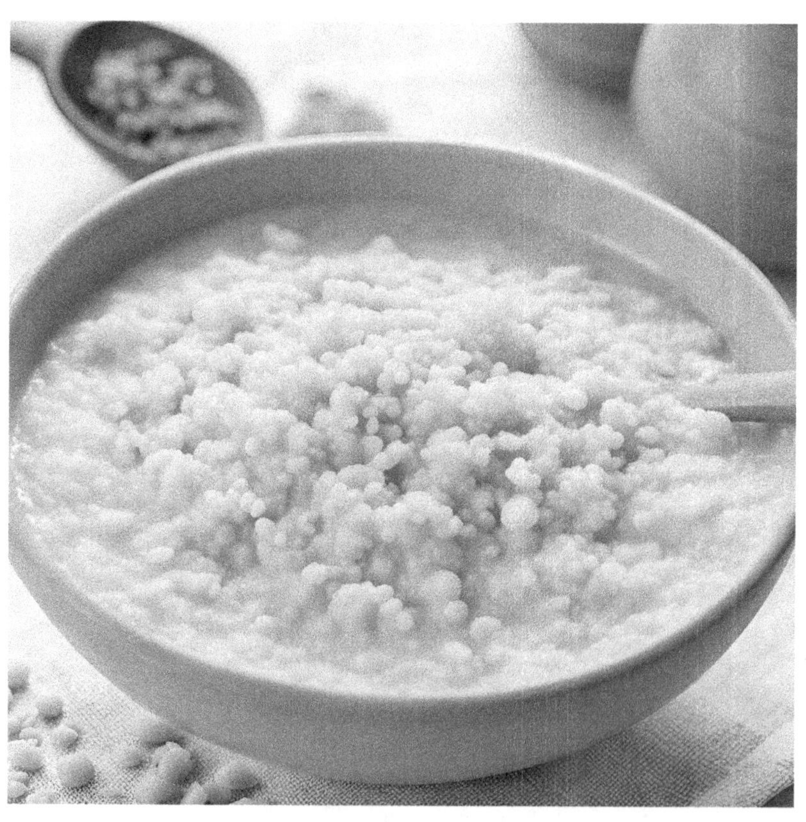

12. Egg White Omelette

Ingredients:

- 4 egg whites
- 1 tbsp olive oil
- 1/2 cup diced bell peppers (green and red)
- 1/4 cup sliced mushrooms
- 1/4 cup diced onions
- Fresh herbs (such as parsley or chives), finely chopped

Instructions:

1. Heat olive oil in a non-stick skillet over medium heat.
2. Sauté bell peppers, mushrooms, and onions until they are soft, about 5 minutes.
3. In a bowl, whisk the egg whites until frothy.
4. Pour the egg whites over the sautéed vegetables in the skillet.
5. Cook until the eggs are set, about 3-4 minutes. Use a spatula to fold the omelette in half.
6. Serve hot, garnished with fresh herbs.

Nutrition Info Per Serving:

- Calories: 140
- Protein: 11g
- Carbohydrates: 5g
- Fat: 8g

Serves: 2
Cooking Time: 10 minutes

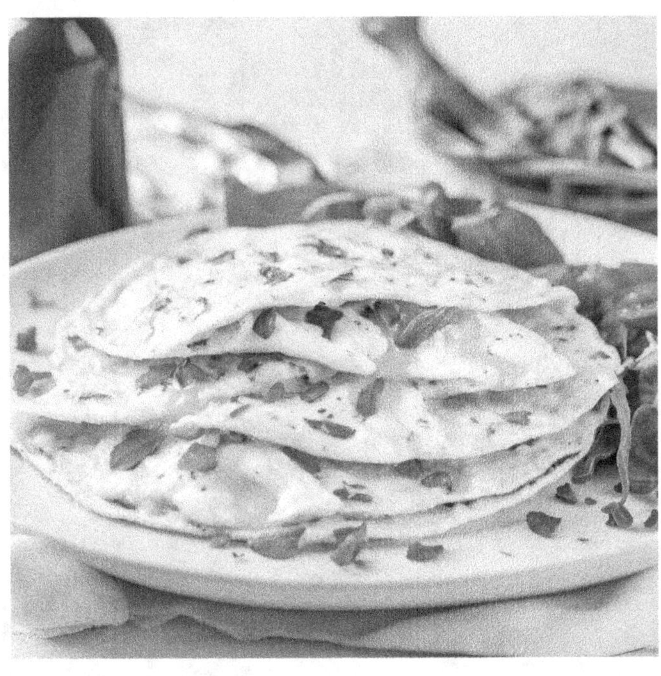

13. Quinoa Breakfast Bowl

Ingredients:

- 1 cup quinoa, rinsed
- 2 cups water
- 1 apple, chopped
- 1/4 cup raisins
- 1/2 tsp cinnamon
- 1 tbsp honey or maple syrup
- 1/4 cup chopped nuts (optional)

Instructions:

1. In a saucepan, combine quinoa and water. Bring to a boil.
2. Reduce heat to low, cover, and simmer for 15 minutes until quinoa is cooked and water is absorbed.
3. Stir in chopped apple, raisins, and cinnamon.
4. Drizzle with honey or maple syrup.
5. Garnish with chopped nuts if using.

Nutrition Info Per Serving:

- Calories: 295
- Protein: 8g
- Carbohydrates: 55g
- Fat: 5g

Serves: 2
Cooking Time: 20 minutes

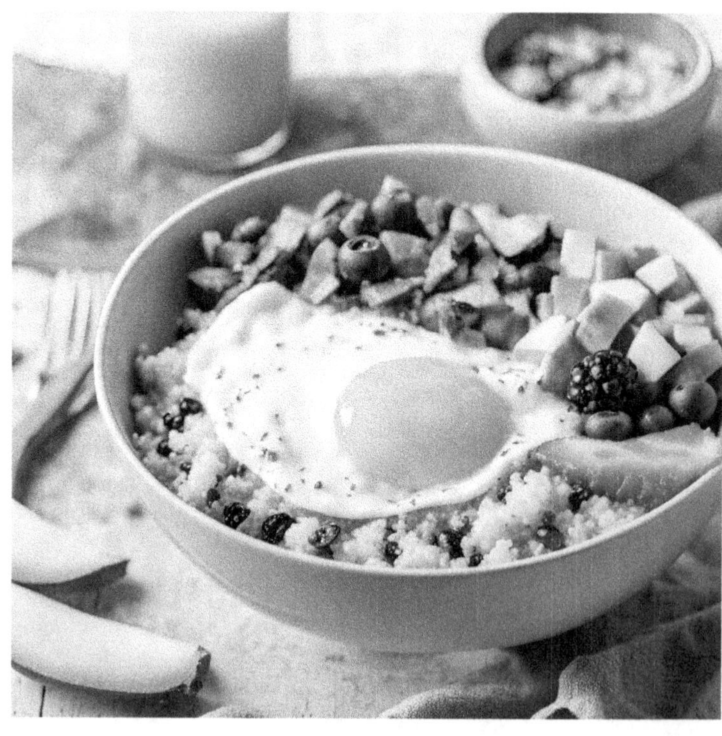

14. Buckwheat Pancakes

Ingredients:

- 1 cup buckwheat flour
- 1 tsp baking powder
- 1 tbsp honey or maple syrup
- 1 cup almond milk
- 1 tbsp olive oil (plus extra for cooking)

Instructions:

1. In a mixing bowl, combine buckwheat flour and baking powder.
2. Stir in honey, almond milk, and olive oil to form a smooth batter.
3. Heat a non-stick pan with a little olive oil over medium heat.
4. Pour batter to form pancakes and cook until bubbles appear, then flip to cook the other side.

Nutrition Info Per Serving:

- Calories: 250
- Protein: 6g
- Carbohydrates: 45g
- Fat: 7g

Serves: 2

Cooking Time: 15 minutes

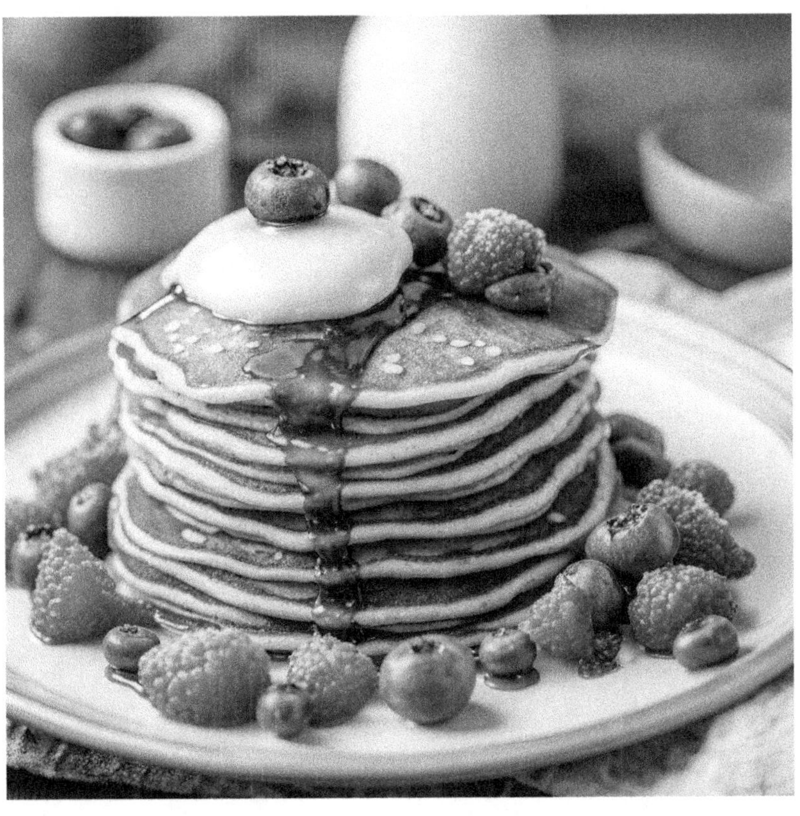

15. Omelette with Fresh Herbs

Ingredients:

- 4 egg whites
- 1 tbsp olive oil
- 1/4 cup chopped fresh herbs (parsley, chives)
- 1/4 cup diced onions

Instructions:

1. Heat olive oil in a non-stick skillet over medium heat.
2. Sauté onions until translucent.
3. Whisk the egg whites and pour over the onions in the skillet.
4. Sprinkle chopped herbs over the egg whites.
5. Cook until the egg whites are set, then fold the omelette in half and serve.

Nutrition Info Per Serving:

- Calories: 130
- Protein: 11g
- Carbohydrates: 3g
- Fat: 8g

Serves: 2

Cooking Time: 10 minutes

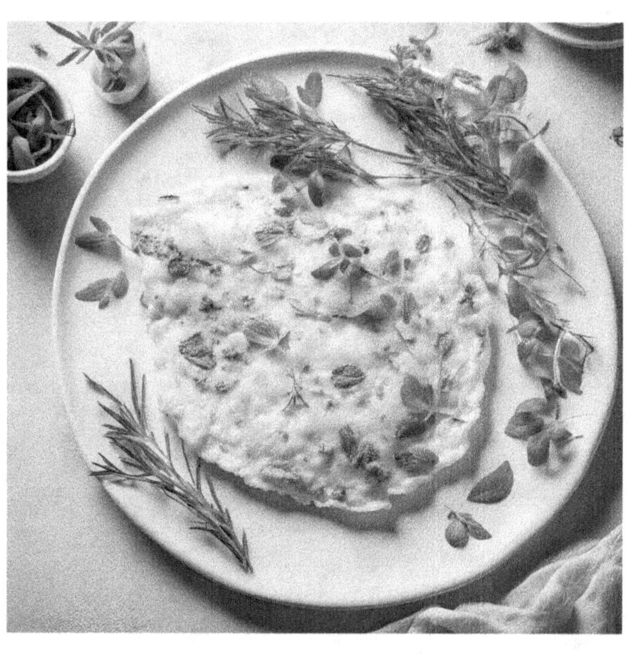

16. Pumpkin Smoothie

Ingredients:

- 1/2 cup pumpkin puree (not pie filling)
- 1 banana
- 1 cup almond milk
- 1 tbsp honey or maple syrup
- 1/2 tsp cinnamon

Instructions:

1. Combine all ingredients in a blender.
2. Blend until smooth.

Nutrition Info Per Serving:

- Calories: 185
- Protein: 2g
- Carbohydrates: 40g
- Fat: 2.5g

Serves: 2
Cooking Time: 5 minutes

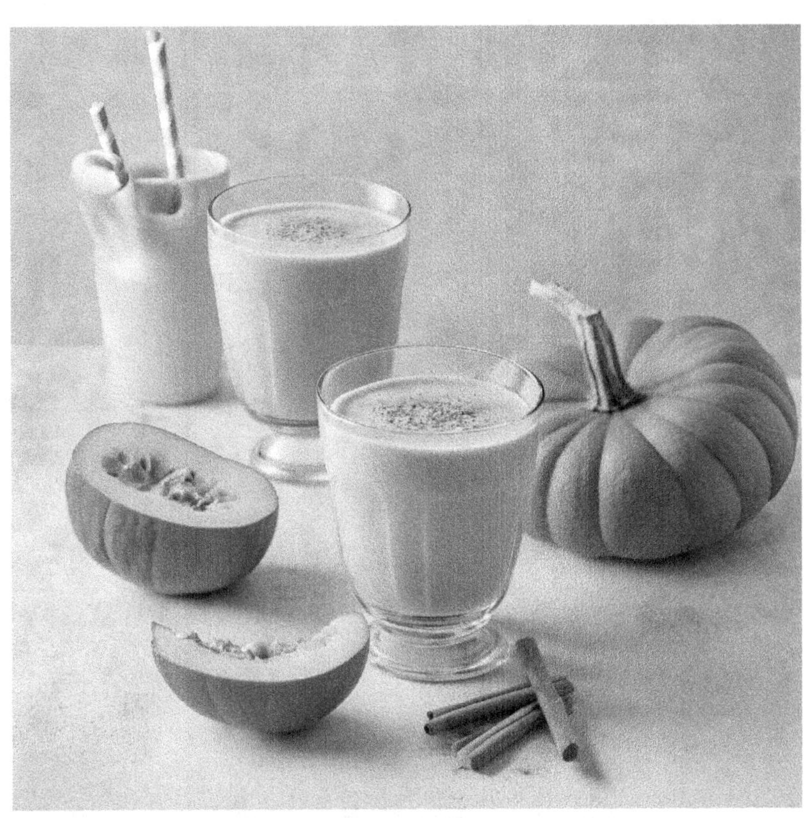

17. Baked Oatmeal

Ingredients:

- 2 cups rolled oats
- 1 apple, chopped
- 1/4 cup raisins
- 2 cups almond milk
- 1 tbsp honey or maple syrup
- 1/2 tsp cinnamon

Instructions:

1. Preheat oven to 375°F (190°C).
2. In a large bowl, mix all ingredients together and transfer to a greased baking dish.
3. Bake for 25 minutes, until set and golden on top.

Nutrition Info Per Serving:

- Calories: 280
- Protein: 6g
- Carbohydrates: 52g
- Fat: 6g

Serves: 4

Cooking Time: 25 minutes

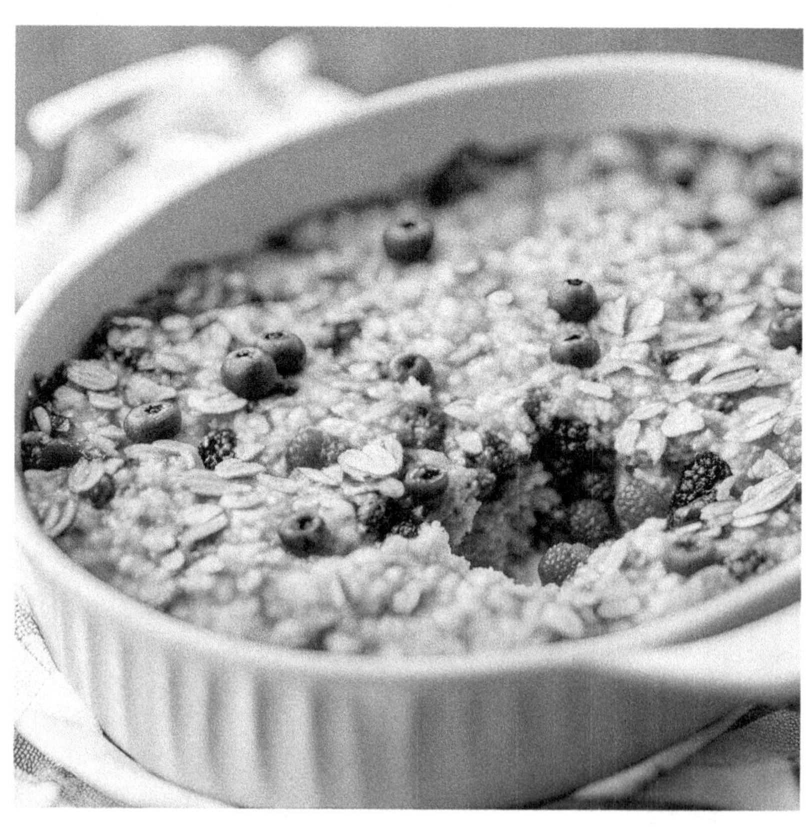

18. Barley Porridge

Ingredients:

- 1 cup pearled barley, rinsed
- 3 cups water
- 1/4 tsp cinnamon
- 1 tbsp honey or maple syrup

Instructions:

1. In a saucepan, combine barley and water. Bring to a boil.
2. Reduce heat to low and simmer until barley is tender and creamy, about 30 minutes.
3. Stir in cinnamon and sweeten with honey or maple syrup.

Nutrition Info Per Serving:

- Calories: 200
- Protein: 4g
- Carbohydrates: 44g
- Fat: 1g

Serves: 4

Cooking Time: 35 minutes

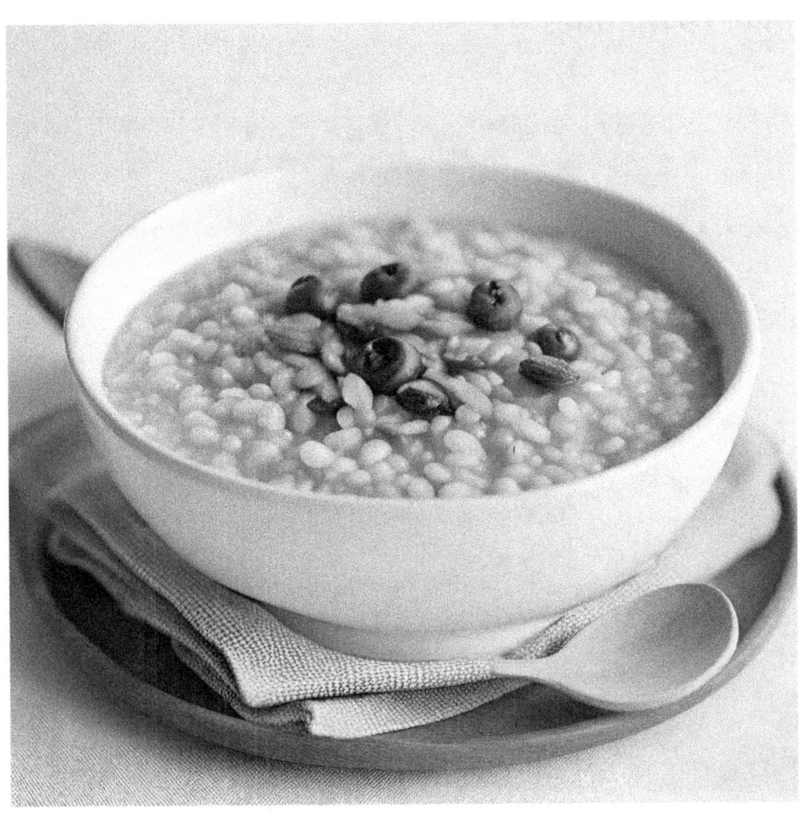

19. Savory Vegetable Pancakes

Ingredients:

- 1 cup grated zucchini
- 1 cup grated carrot
- 1/2 cup buckwheat flour
- 1 egg, beaten
- 1 tbsp olive oil (for cooking)

Instructions:

1. Combine zucchini, carrot, buckwheat flour, and egg in a bowl and mix well.
2. Heat olive oil in a skillet over medium heat.
3. Scoop the vegetable mixture into the skillet, flattening to form pancakes.
4. Cook until golden brown on both sides.

Nutrition Info Per Serving:

- Calories: 120
- Protein: 4g
- Carbohydrates: 18g
- Fat: 4g

Serves: 4

Cooking Time: 20 minutes

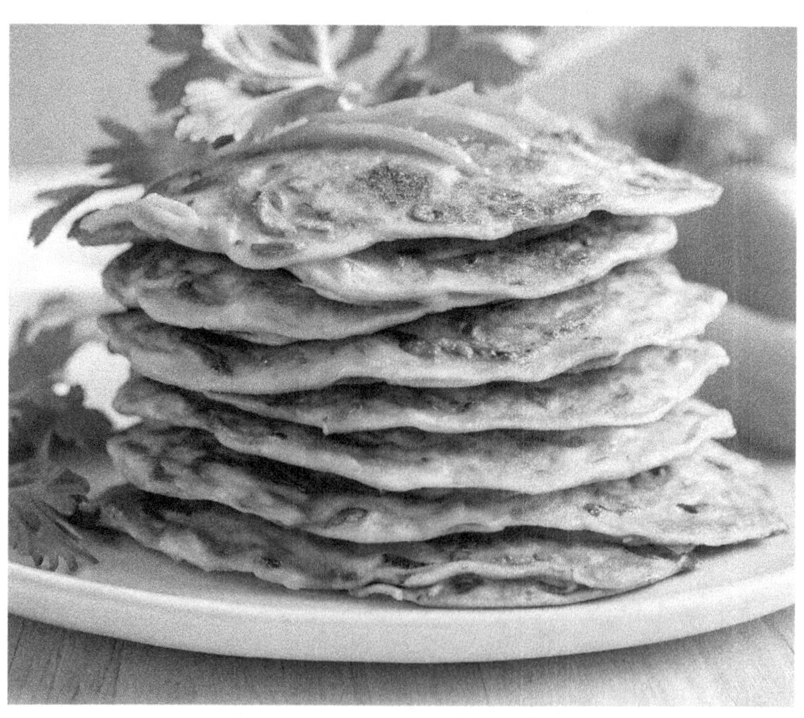

20. Vanilla Almond Milk Porridge

Ingredients:

- 1 cup rolled oats
- 2 cups almond milk
- 1 tsp vanilla extract
- 1 tbsp honey or maple syrup

Instructions:

1. In a saucepan, bring almond milk to a boil.
2. Add oats and reduce heat to simmer.
3. Cook until oats are tender, about 5 minutes.
4. Stir in vanilla extract and honey or maple syrup.

Nutrition Info Per Serving:

- Calories: 210
- Protein: 5g
- Carbohydrates: 38g
- Fat: 4g

Serves: 2
Cooking Time: 10 minutes

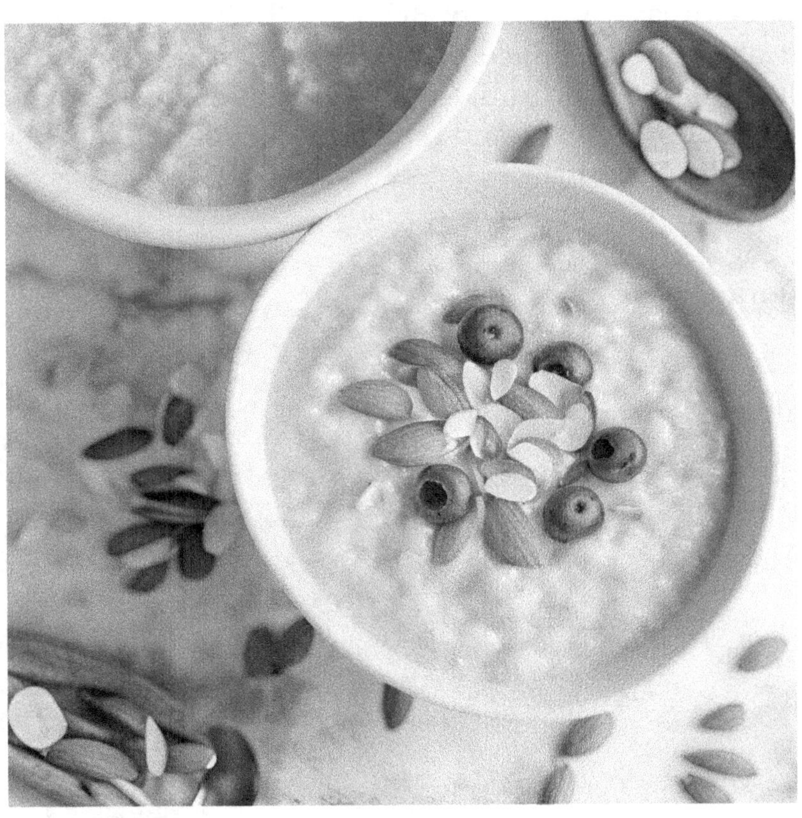

Lunch Recipes

1. Chicken and Rice Soup

Ingredients:
- 2 chicken breasts, skinless and boneless
- 1 cup rice, rinsed
- 6 cups low-sodium chicken broth
- 1 cup chopped carrots
- 1 cup chopped celery
- 1/2 cup chopped onions
- 1 tsp thyme
- 1 tbsp olive oil

Instructions:
1. In a large pot, heat olive oil over medium heat. Sauté onions, carrots, and celery until soft.
2. Add chicken breasts and broth. Bring to a boil.
3. Add rice and thyme. Reduce heat to a simmer.
4. Cook for 25 minutes, or until the rice and chicken are fully cooked.
5. Remove chicken, shred it, and return to the pot.

Nutrition Info Per Serving:
- Calories: 320
- Protein: 26g
- Carbohydrates: 40g
- Fat: 8g

Serves: 4
Cooking Time: 35 minutes

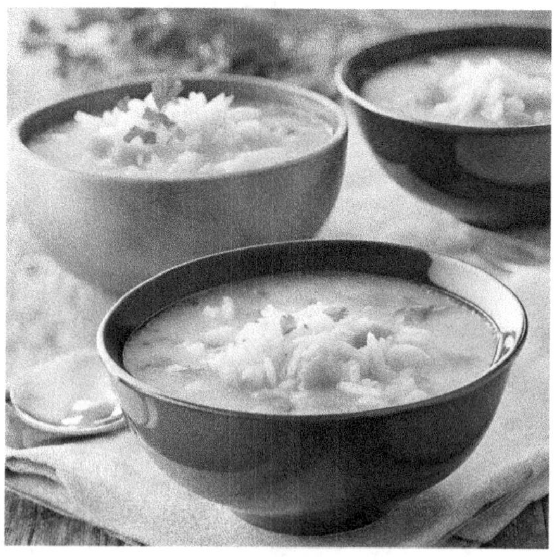

2. Turkey Sandwich

Ingredients:

- 4 slices whole wheat bread
- 8 oz sliced turkey breast
- 2 tbsp mayonnaise
- 1/4 cup shredded lettuce
- 1/2 cucumber, sliced

Instructions:

1. Spread mayonnaise on each slice of bread.
2. Layer the turkey, cucumber, and lettuce on two slices of bread.
3. Top with the remaining slices to form sandwiches.

Nutrition Info Per Serving:

- Calories: 300
- Protein: 20g
- Carbohydrates: 30g
- Fat: 12g

Serves: 2

Cooking Time: 5 minutes

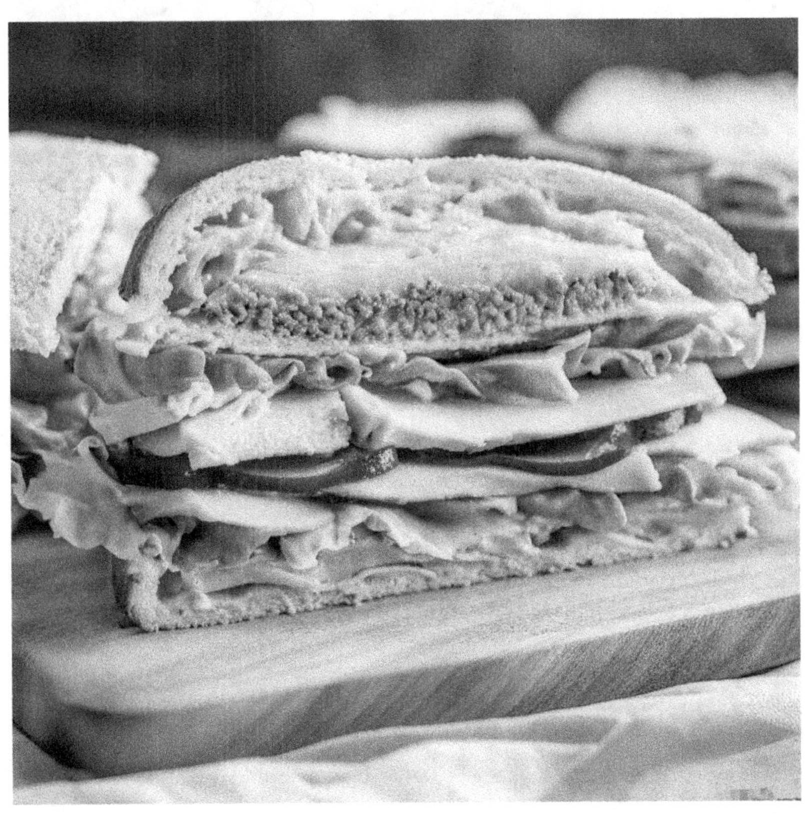

3. Cucumber and Dill Salad
Ingredients:
- 2 large cucumbers, peeled and thinly sliced
- 1/4 cup fresh dill, chopped
- 2 tbsp olive oil
- 1 tbsp white vinegar

Instructions:
1. In a salad bowl, combine cucumbers and dill.
2. Drizzle with olive oil and vinegar, and toss gently to coat.

Nutrition Info Per Serving:
- Calories: 100
- Protein: 1g
- Carbohydrates: 8g
- Fat: 7g

Serves: 4
Cooking Time: 5 minutes

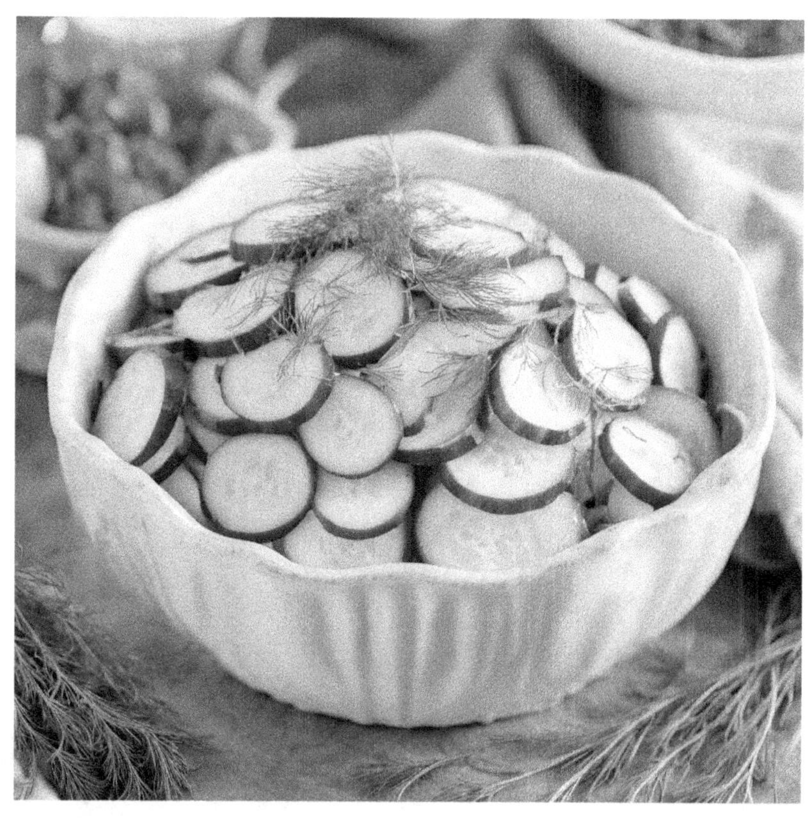

4. Roasted Chicken Breast

Ingredients:

- 4 chicken breasts, skinless and boneless
- 1 tbsp olive oil
- 1 tsp garlic powder
- 1 tsp dried parsley
- 1/4 tsp thyme

Instructions:

1. Preheat oven to 375°F (190°C).
2. Rub each chicken breast with olive oil and sprinkle with garlic powder, parsley, and thyme.
3. Place in a baking dish and roast for 25-30 minutes, until fully cooked.

Nutrition Info Per Serving:

- Calories: 165
- Protein: 25g
- Carbohydrates: 0g
- Fat: 7g

Serves: 4Cooking Time: 30 minutes

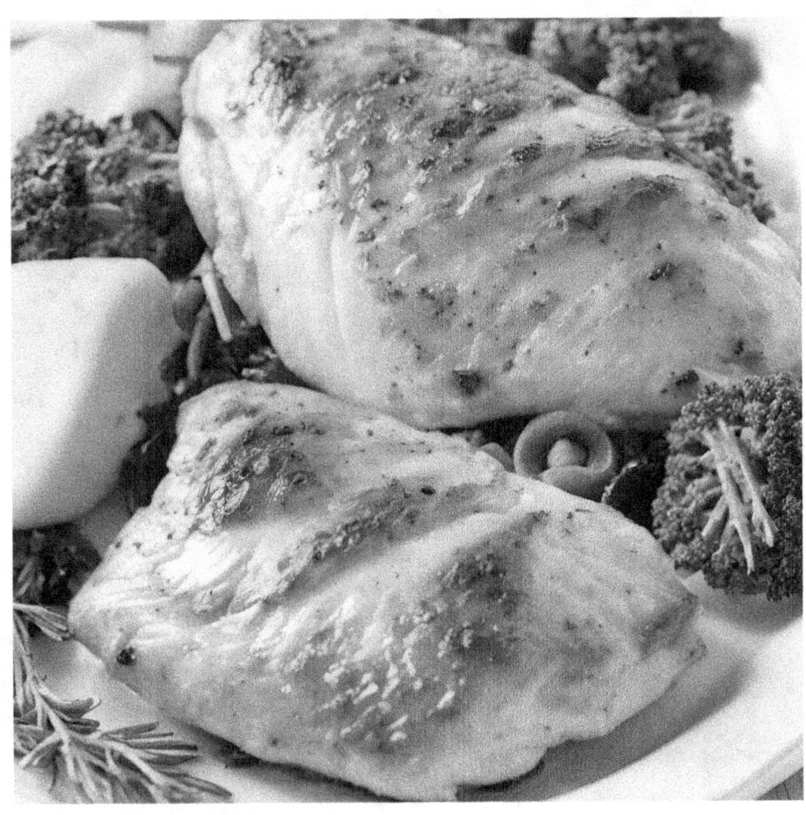

5. Pasta with Olive Oil and Garlic

Ingredients:

- 8 oz pasta (e.g., spaghetti)
- 3 tbsp olive oil
- 3 cloves garlic, minced
- Fresh herbs (such as parsley), chopped

Instructions:

1. Cook pasta according to package instructions until al dente.
2. In a pan, heat olive oil over medium heat and sauté garlic until fragrant.
3. Toss cooked pasta with garlic oil and fresh herbs.

Nutrition Info Per Serving:

- Calories: 350
- Protein: 10g
- Carbohydrates: 56g
- Fat: 10g

Serves: 4Cooking Time: 20 minutes

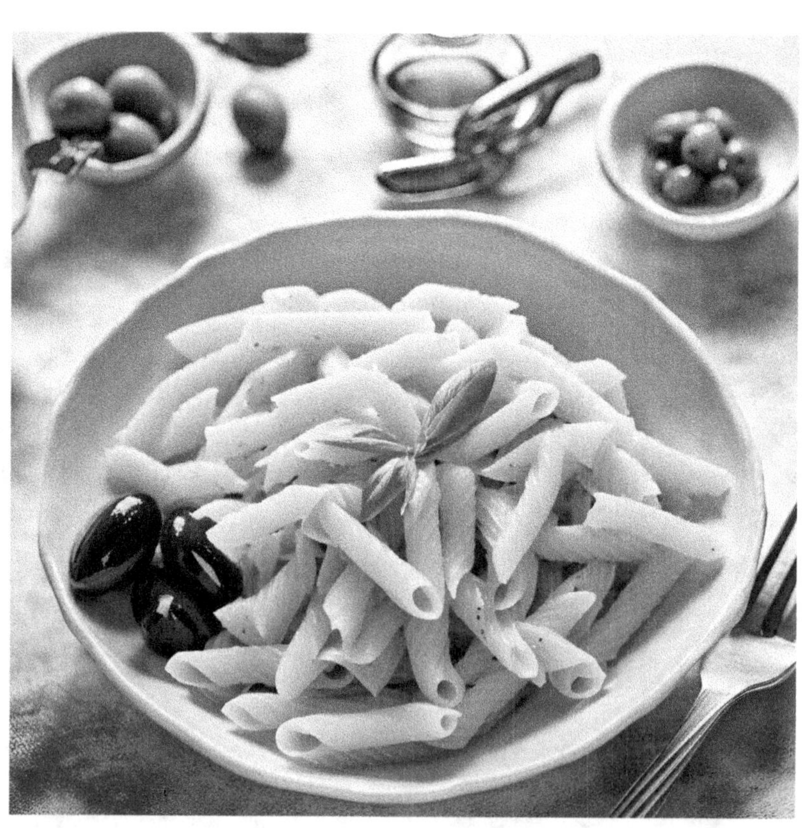

6. Beef Stew

Ingredients:

- 1 lb beef stew meat, cut into cubes
- 3 cups beef broth
- 1 cup diced carrots
- 1 cup diced potatoes
- 1/2 cup diced celery
- 1 tsp thyme
- 1 tbsp olive oil

Instructions:

1. In a large pot, heat olive oil over medium heat. Brown the beef cubes.
2. Add broth, carrots, potatoes, celery, and thyme.
3. Bring to a boil, then simmer for about 1 hour until meat is tender.

Nutrition Info Per Serving:

- Calories: 350
- Protein: 24g
- Carbohydrates: 25g
- Fat: 18g

Serves: 4Cooking Time: 75 minutes

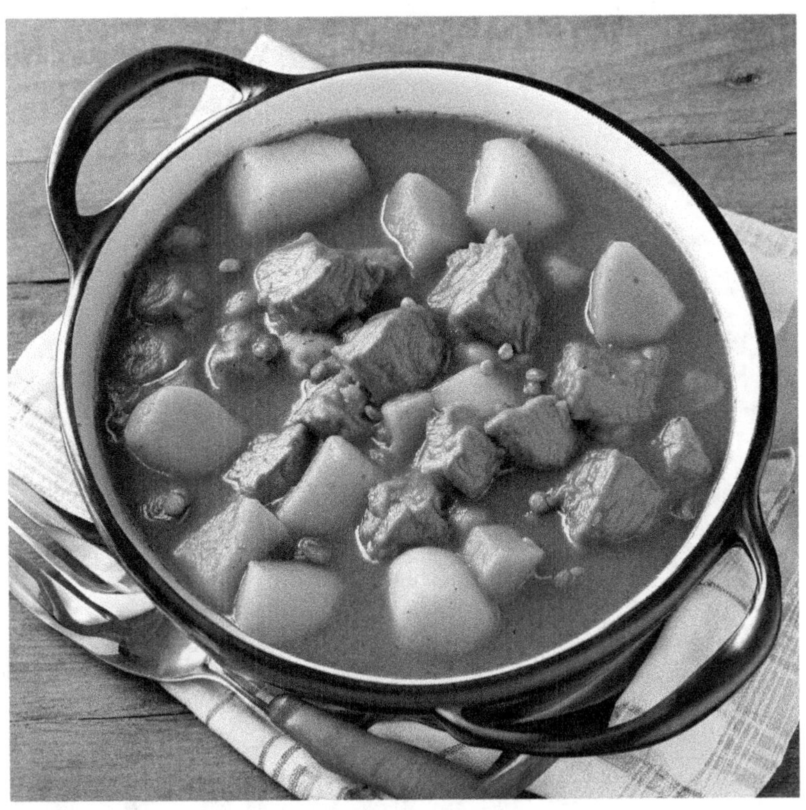

7. Quinoa Salad

Ingredients:

- 1 cup quinoa, rinsed
- 2 cups water
- 1/2 cup diced cucumber
- 1/2 cup diced bell pepper
- 1/4 cup chopped fresh parsley
- 2 tbsp olive oil
- 1 tbsp white vinegar

Instructions:

1. In a saucepan, bring water to a boil. Add quinoa and reduce to a simmer. Cook for 15 minutes.
2. Fluff quinoa with a fork and let cool.
3. Add cucumber, bell pepper, and parsley to the quinoa.
4. Dress with olive oil and vinegar, and toss to combine.

Nutrition Info Per Serving:

- Calories: 250
- Protein: 8g
- Carbohydrates: 35g
- Fat: 9g

Serves: 4

Cooking Time: 20 minutes

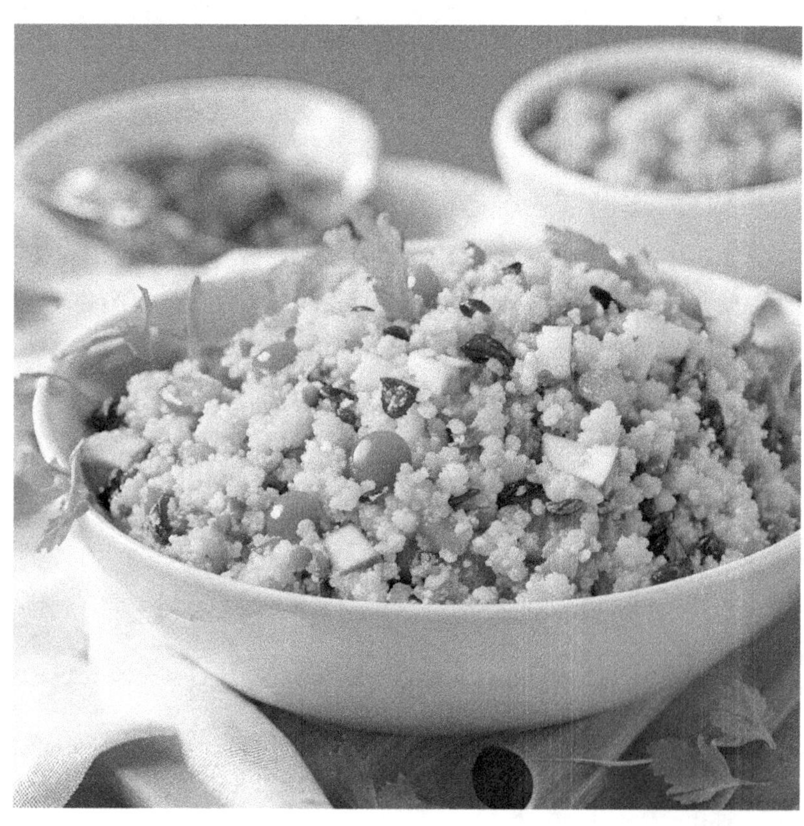

8. Baked Potato with Chives

Ingredients:

- 4 large potatoes
- 1 tbsp olive oil
- 2 tbsp chopped chives

Instructions:

1. Preheat oven to 400°F (200°C).
2. Pierce potatoes with a fork, rub with olive oil, and wrap in foil.
3. Bake for 1 hour until tender.
4. Sprinkle with chives before serving.

Nutrition Info Per Serving:

- Calories: 210
- Protein: 4g
- Carbohydrates: 40g
- Fat: 5g

Serves: 4

Cooking Time: 60 minutes

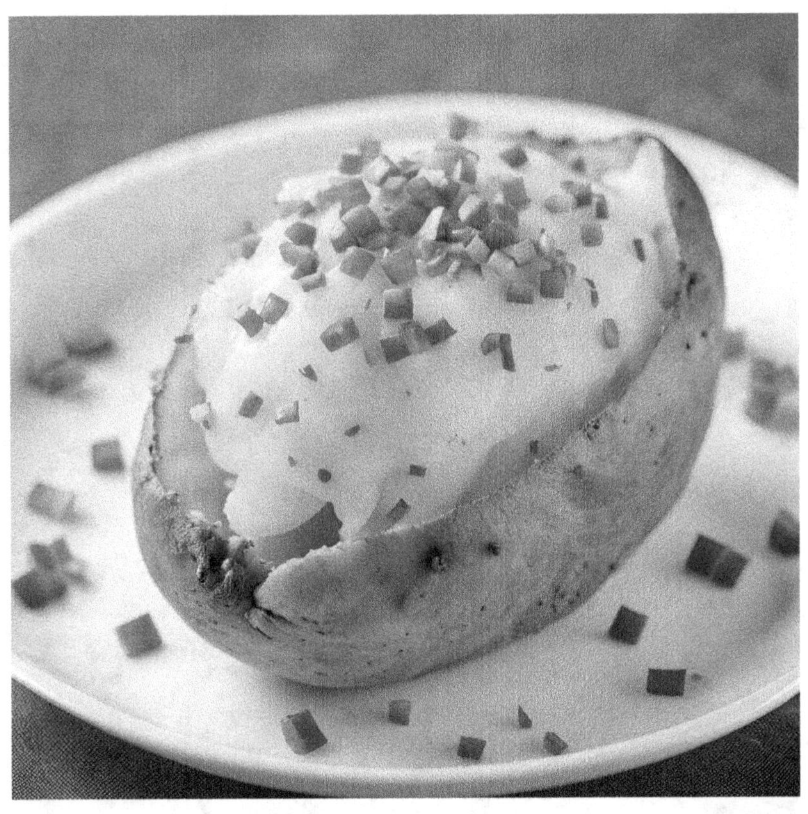

9. Spinach and Cheese Quesadilla

Ingredients:

- 4 whole wheat tortillas
- 1 cup shredded mozzarella cheese
- 1 cup fresh spinach, chopped
- 1 tbsp olive oil

Instructions:

1. Heat a non-stick skillet over medium heat.
2. Place a tortilla in the skillet, sprinkle half with cheese and spinach.
3. Fold tortilla over and cook until golden on both sides.

Nutrition Info Per Serving:

- Calories: 250
- Protein: 12g
- Carbohydrates: 22g
- Fat: 14g

Serves: 4

Cooking Time: 10 minutes

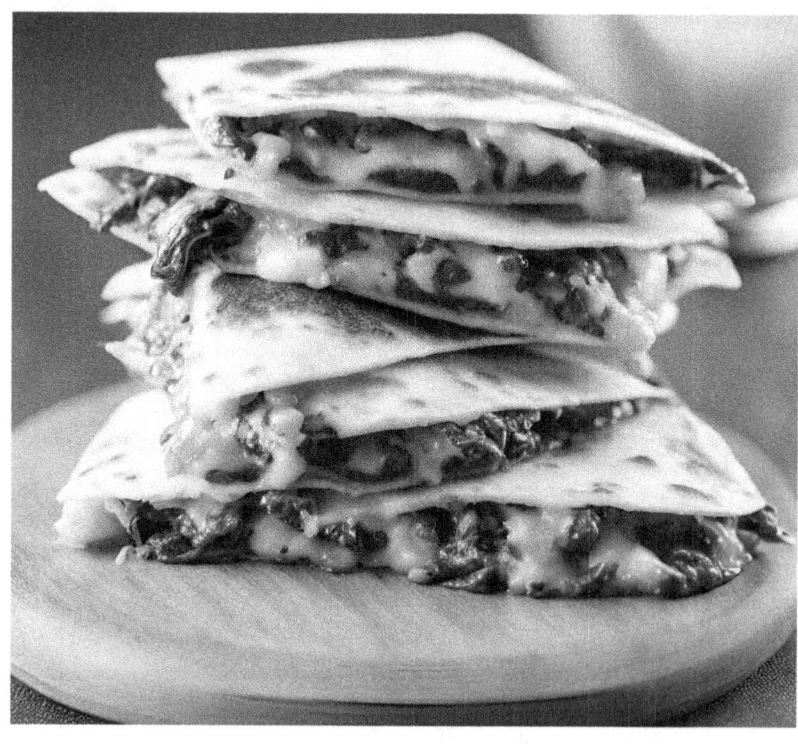

10. Mild White Fish Tacos

Ingredients:

- 8 oz white fish fillets (e.g., tilapia)
- 8 small corn tortillas
- 1 cup shredded lettuce
- 1/2 cup diced cucumber
- 1 tbsp olive oil

Instructions:

1. Heat olive oil in a pan over medium heat. Cook fish until opaque and flaky.
2. Warm tortillas in a dry skillet.
3. Place fish, lettuce, and cucumber in tortillas and serve.

Nutrition Info Per Serving:

- Calories: 220
- Protein: 14g
- Carbohydrates: 24g
- Fat: 8g

Serves: 4Cooking Time: 15 minutes

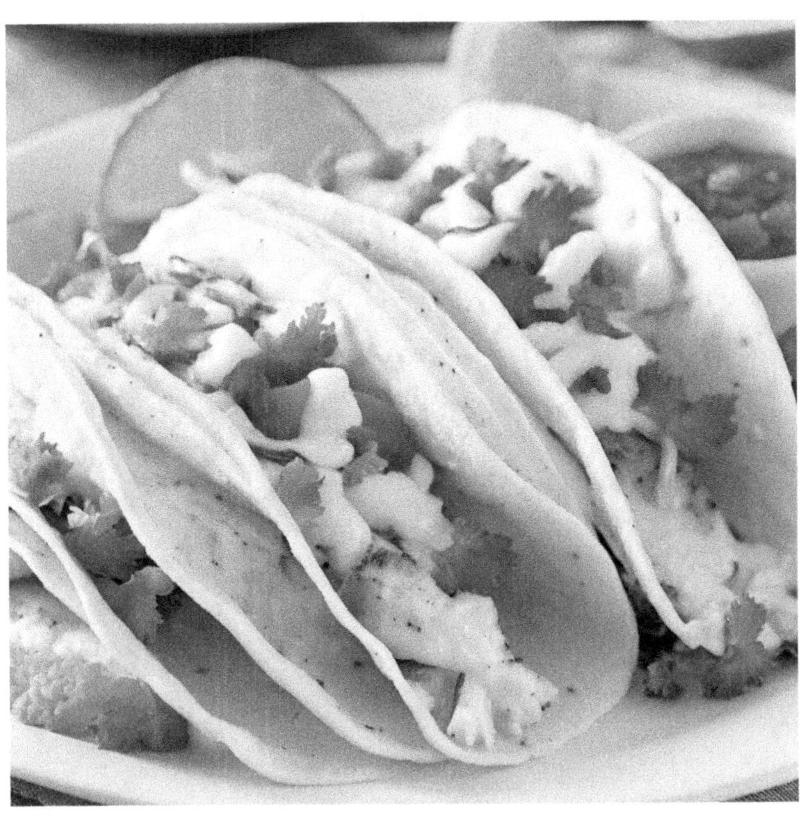

11. Chicken Salad

Ingredients:

- 2 cups cooked chicken breast, chopped
- 1/4 cup mayonnaise
- 1/4 cup plain Greek yogurt
- 1/2 cup diced celery
- 1/4 cup chopped almonds
- 1/4 tsp dried dill

Instructions:

1. In a large bowl, combine the chicken, mayonnaise, Greek yogurt, celery, almonds, and dill.
2. Mix well until all ingredients are evenly distributed.
3. Chill in the refrigerator before serving to enhance the flavors.

Nutrition Info Per Serving:

- Calories: 290
- Protein: 27g
- Carbohydrates: 4g
- Fat: 18g

Serves: 4

Cooking Time: 10 minutes

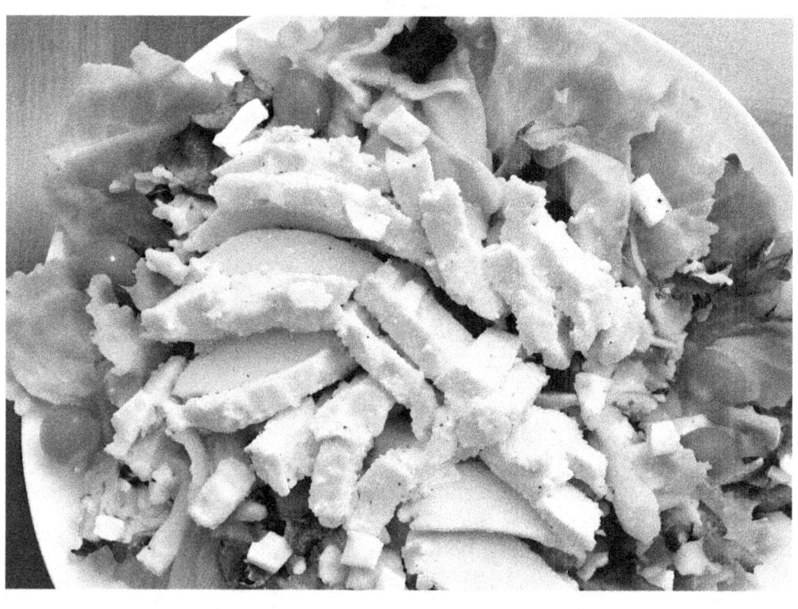

12. Vegetable and Barley Soup

Ingredients:

- 1/2 cup pearl barley, rinsed
- 1 liter vegetable broth
- 1 cup diced carrots
- 1 cup diced celery
- 1 cup chopped leeks
- 1 tbsp olive oil
- 1 tsp thyme

Instructions:

1. In a large pot, heat the olive oil over medium heat. Add leeks, carrots, and celery; sauté until softened.
2. Add the vegetable broth and barley; bring to a boil.
3. Reduce heat to a simmer, cover, and cook for about 1 hour until the barley is tender.
4. Add thyme in the last 10 minutes of cooking.

Nutrition Info Per Serving:

- Calories: 150
- Protein: 4g
- Carbohydrates: 30g
- Fat: 3g

Serves: 4

Cooking Time: 70 minutes

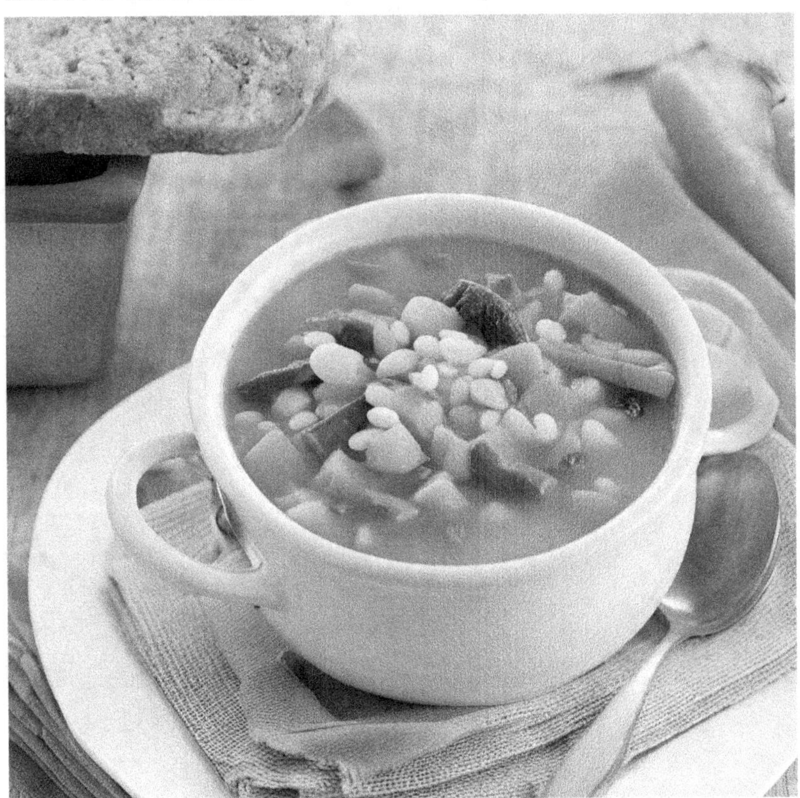

13. Turkey Meatloaf

Ingredients:

- 1 lb ground turkey
- 1 egg
- 1/2 cup breadcrumbs
- 1/4 cup milk
- 1/2 cup chopped onions
- 1 tsp dried thyme

Instructions:

1. Preheat oven to 375°F (190°C).
2. In a bowl, mix all ingredients until well combined.
3. Press the mixture into a loaf pan.
4. Bake for 45 minutes, or until cooked through.

Nutrition Info Per Serving:

- Calories: 240
- Protein: 28g
- Carbohydrates: 12g
- Fat: 10g

Serves: 4

Cooking Time: 45 minutes

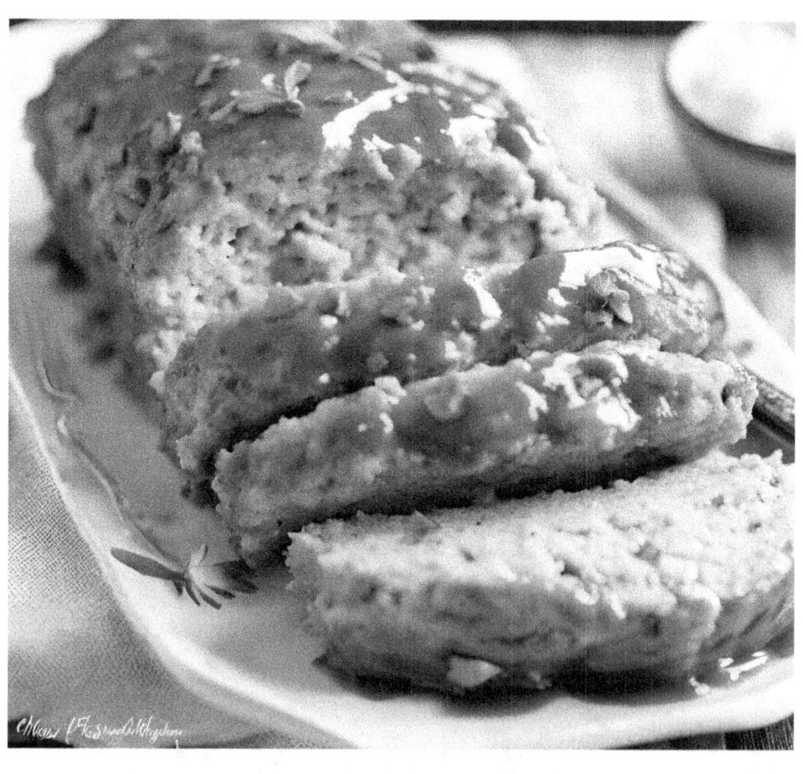

14. Egg Salad
Ingredients:

- 6 hard-boiled eggs, chopped
- 1/4 cup mayonnaise
- 1/4 cup plain Greek yogurt
- 1 tbsp chopped chives
- 1 tsp mustard

Instructions:

1. In a bowl, combine eggs, mayonnaise, Greek yogurt, chives, and mustard.
2. Stir until well mixed.
3. Refrigerate before serving to blend flavors.

Nutrition Info Per Serving:

- Calories: 230
- Protein: 13g
- Carbohydrates: 2g
- Fat: 18g

Serves: 4
Cooking Time: 10 minutes

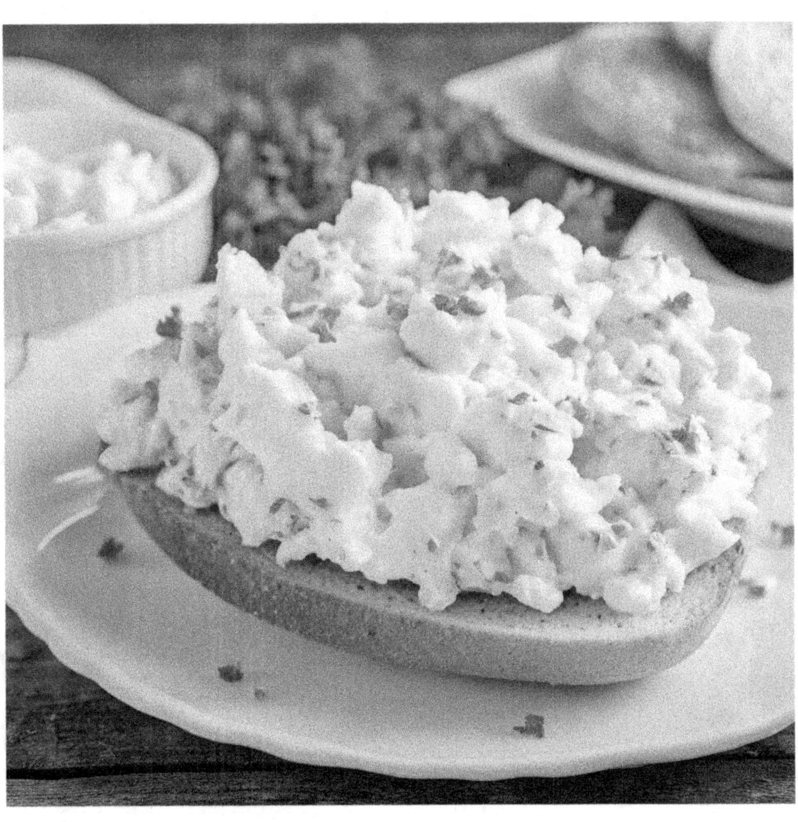

15. Sautéed Green Beans with Almonds

Ingredients:

- 2 cups green beans, trimmed
- 1 tbsp olive oil
- 1/4 cup sliced almonds
- 1 tsp garlic powder

Instructions:

1. Heat olive oil in a skillet over medium heat.
2. Add green beans and sauté until tender-crisp, about 5 minutes.
3. Stir in sliced almonds and garlic powder, cook for an additional 2 minutes.

Nutrition Info Per Serving:

- Calories: 100
- Protein: 3g
- Carbohydrates: 8g
- Fat: 7g

Serves: 4

Cooking Time: 7 minutes

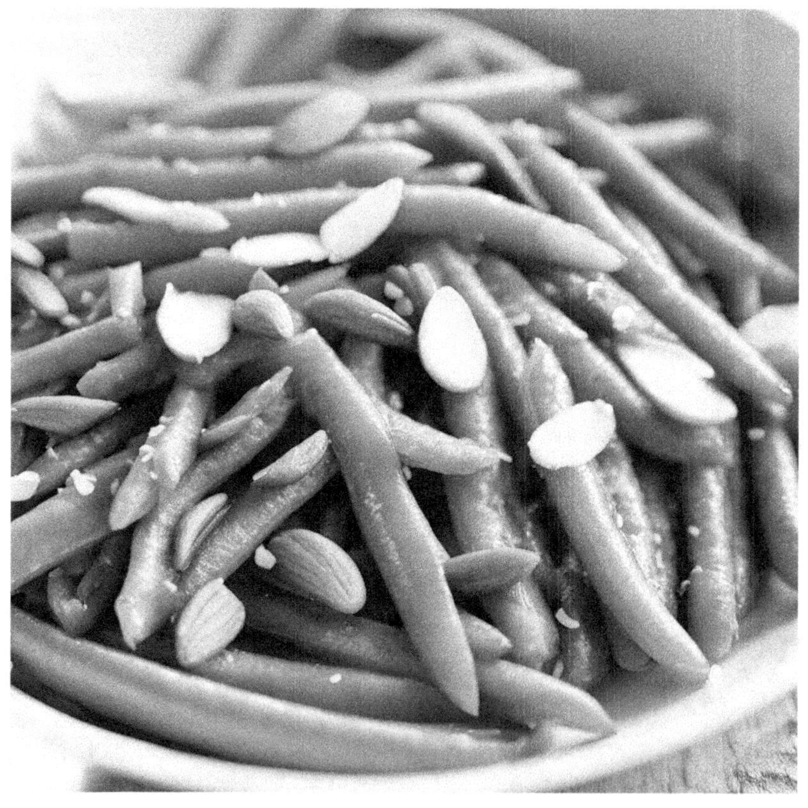

16. Mushroom and Leek Pasta

Ingredients:

- 8 oz pasta
- 1 tbsp olive oil
- 1 cup chopped leeks
- 1 cup sliced mushrooms
- 1/4 cup cream
- Fresh herbs (parsley or thyme), chopped

Instructions:

1. Cook pasta according to package directions until al dente.
2. In a skillet, heat olive oil over medium heat. Sauté leeks and mushrooms until tender.
3. Add cooked pasta and cream to the skillet. Toss to coat.
4. Garnish with fresh herbs.

Nutrition Info Per Serving:

- Calories: 300
- Protein: 10g
- Carbohydrates: 45g
- Fat: 10g

Serves: 4
Cooking Time: 20 minutes

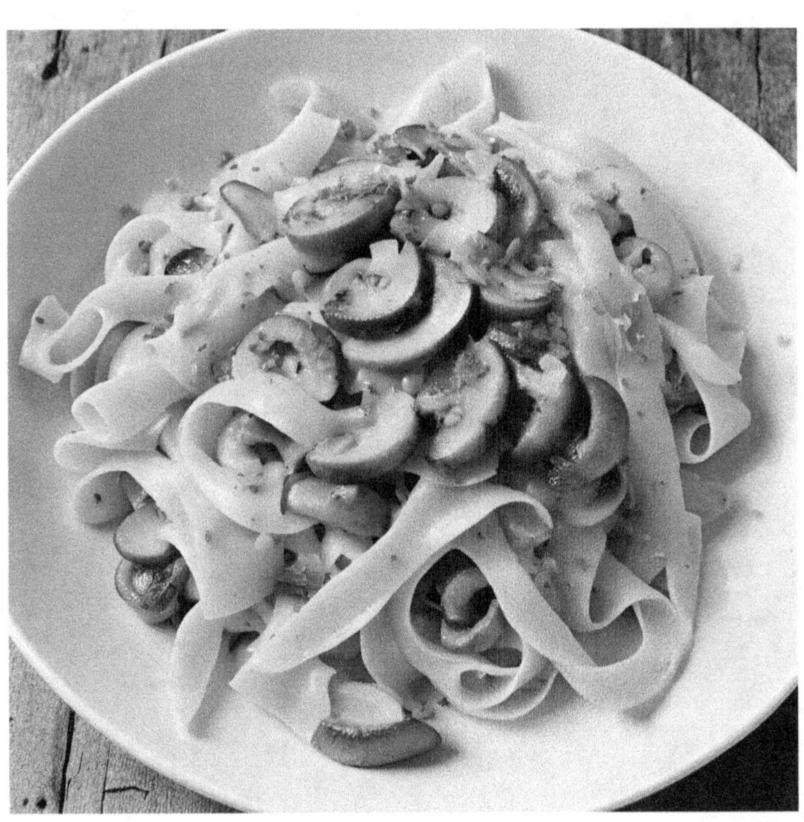

17. Grilled Cheese Sandwich

Ingredients:

- 8 slices whole wheat bread
- 4 slices cheddar cheese
- 2 tbsp butter

Instructions:

1. Butter one side of each bread slice.
2. Place a slice of cheese between two slices of bread, buttered sides out.
3. Heat a skillet over medium heat and grill each sandwich until golden brown on both sides.

Nutrition Info Per Serving:

- Calories: 350
- Protein: 16g
- Carbohydrates: 30g
- Fat: 20g

Serves: 4

Cooking Time: 10 minutes

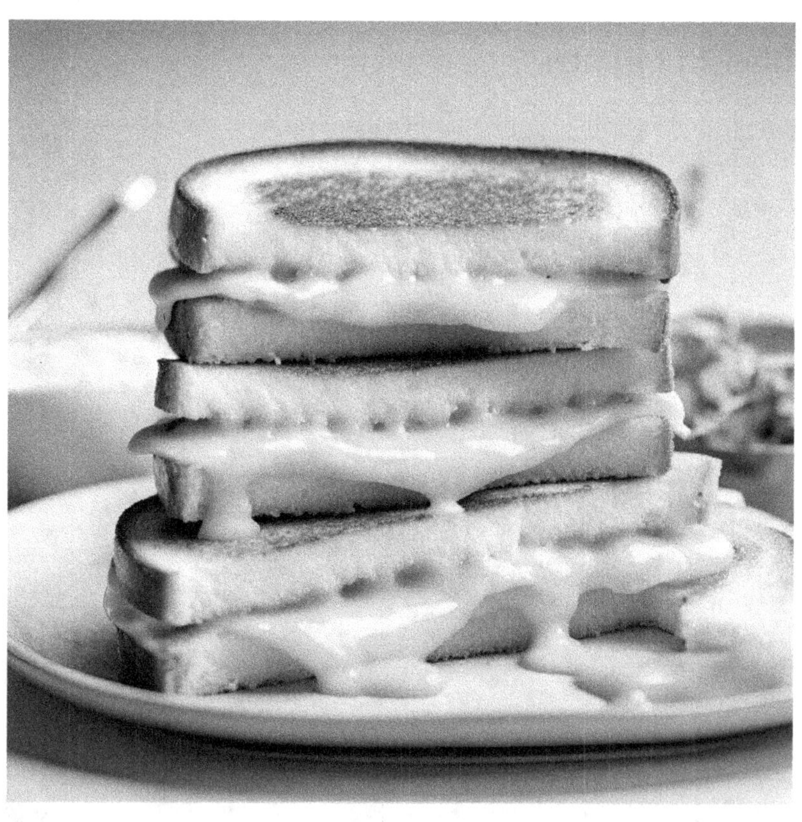

18. Pasta Primavera

Ingredients:

- 8 oz pasta
- 1 tbsp olive oil
- 1 cup chopped bell peppers
- 1 cup broccoli florets
- 1/2 cup peas
- 1/4 cup cream
- Fresh herbs (basil or parsley), chopped

Instructions:

1. Cook pasta according to package directions until al dente.
2. In a large skillet, heat olive oil over medium heat. Sauté bell peppers, broccoli, and peas until tender.
3. Add cooked pasta and cream to the skillet. Toss to combine.
4. Garnish with fresh herbs.

Nutrition Info Per Serving:

- Calories: 320
- Protein: 10g
- Carbohydrates: 45g
- Fat: 11g

Serves: 4
Cooking Time: 20 minutes

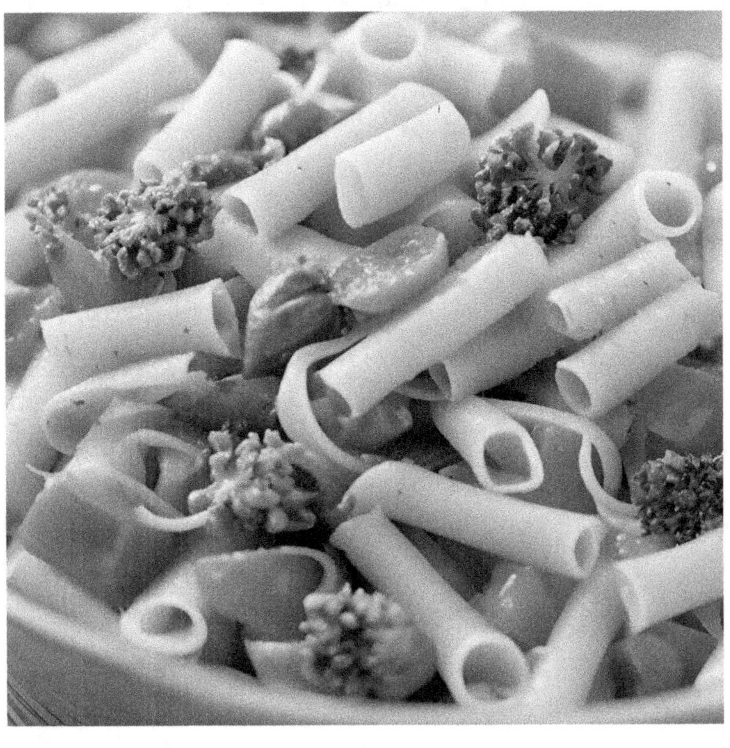

19. Roasted Turkey and Sweet Potato
Ingredients:
- 1 lb turkey breast
- 2 large sweet potatoes, peeled and cubed
- 1 tbsp olive oil
- 1 tsp dried rosemary

Instructions:
1. Preheat oven to 375°F (190°C).
2. Place turkey and sweet potatoes on a baking sheet. Drizzle with olive oil and sprinkle with rosemary.
3. Roast for 45 minutes, or until turkey is cooked through and sweet potatoes are tender.

Nutrition Info Per Serving:
- Calories: 290
- Protein: 30g
- Carbohydrates: 28g
- Fat: 8g

Serves: 4
Cooking Time: 45 minutes

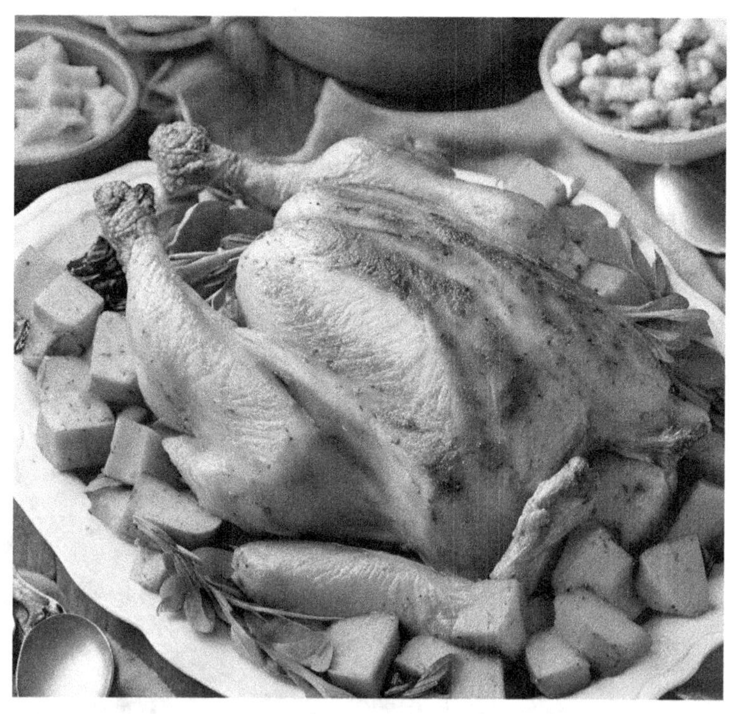

20. Creamy Polenta with Mushrooms

Ingredients:

- 1 cup polenta
- 4 cups water
- 1/2 cup cream
- 1 cup sliced mushrooms
- 1 tbsp olive oil
- Fresh herbs (thyme), chopped

Instructions:

1. Bring water to a boil in a saucepan. Gradually whisk in polenta.
2. Reduce heat to low and cook, stirring frequently, until polenta is thickened, about 30 minutes.
3. In a separate skillet, heat olive oil over medium heat. Sauté mushrooms until golden.
4. Stir cream and sautéed mushrooms into the cooked polenta. Garnish with fresh herbs.

Nutrition Info Per Serving:

- Calories: 270
- Protein: 5g
- Carbohydrates: 38g
- Fat: 11g

Serves: 4
Cooking Time: 40 minutes

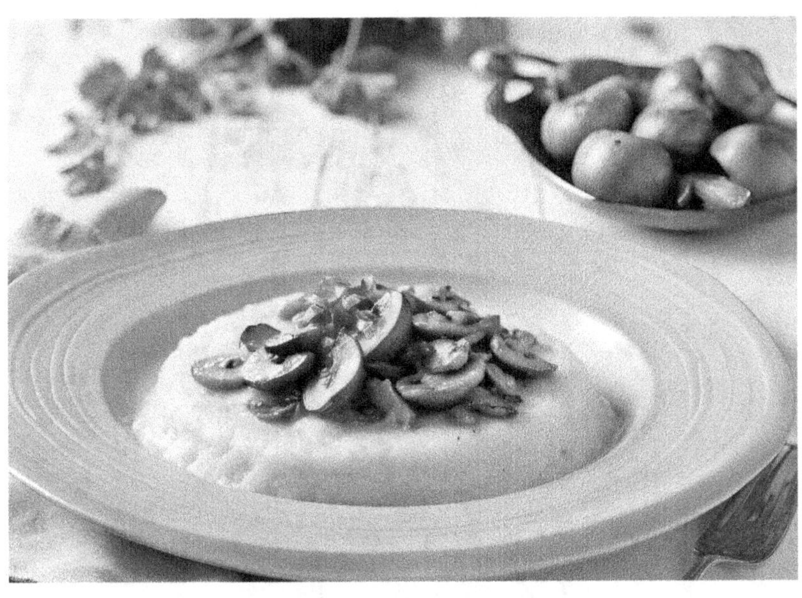

Dinner Recipes

1. Herb-Roasted Turkey Breast
Ingredients:
- 2 lbs turkey breast
- 2 tbsp olive oil
- 1 tsp dried thyme
- 1 tsp dried rosemary
- 1 tsp dried sage
- 1/2 tsp garlic powder

Instructions:
1. Preheat oven to 350°F (175°C).
2. Rub the turkey breast with olive oil.
3. Mix thyme, rosemary, sage, and garlic powder together, then rub onto the turkey.
4. Place the turkey in a roasting pan and roast for about 1-1.5 hours, or until the internal temperature reaches 165°F (74°C).
5. Let rest for 10 minutes before slicing.

Nutrition Info Per Serving:
- Calories: 190
- Protein: 35g
- Carbohydrates: 0g
- Fat: 5g

Serves: 4
Cooking Time: 90 minutes

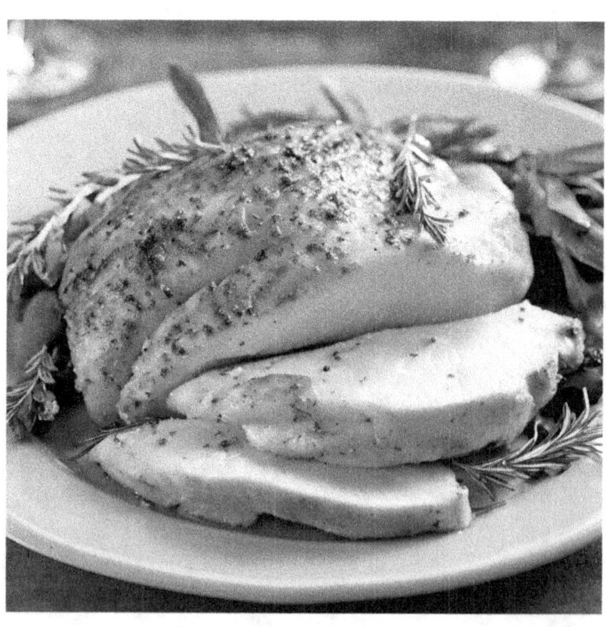

2. Maple Glazed Salmon

Ingredients:

- 4 salmon fillets (6 oz each)
- 2 tbsp olive oil
- 3 tbsp maple syrup
- 1/2 tsp garlic powder
- 1/2 tsp dried dill

Instructions:

1. Preheat the oven to 400°F (200°C).
2. In a small bowl, mix maple syrup, olive oil, garlic powder, and dill.
3. Place salmon fillets on a baking sheet lined with parchment paper.
4. Brush each fillet with the maple mixture.
5. Bake for about 15-20 minutes, or until salmon flakes easily with a fork.

Nutrition Info Per Serving:

- Calories: 350
- Protein: 23g
- Carbohydrates: 11g
- Fat: 23g

Serves: 4
Cooking Time: 20 minutes

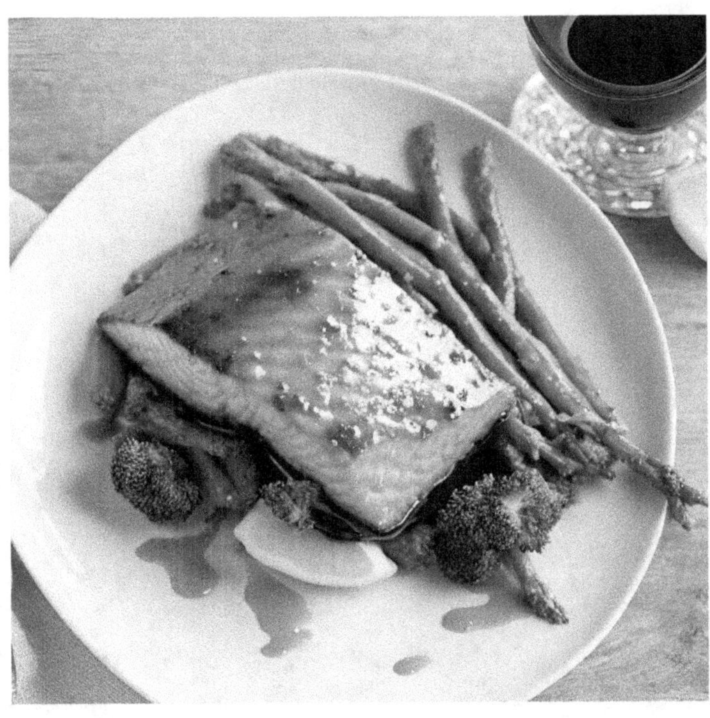

3. Beef Sirloin with Parsley

Ingredients:

- 2 lbs beef sirloin, cut into 4 steaks
- 2 tbsp olive oil
- 1/2 cup chopped fresh parsley
- 1 tsp garlic powder
- 1 tsp dried oregano

Instructions:

1. Preheat the grill to medium-high heat.
2. Rub each steak with olive oil, garlic powder, and oregano.
3. Grill steaks for about 4-5 minutes per side for medium-rare, or to desired doneness.
4. Once done, garnish with fresh chopped parsley.

Nutrition Info Per Serving:

- Calories: 400
- Protein: 45g
- Carbohydrates: 1g
- Fat: 24g

Serves: 4

Cooking Time: 20 minutes

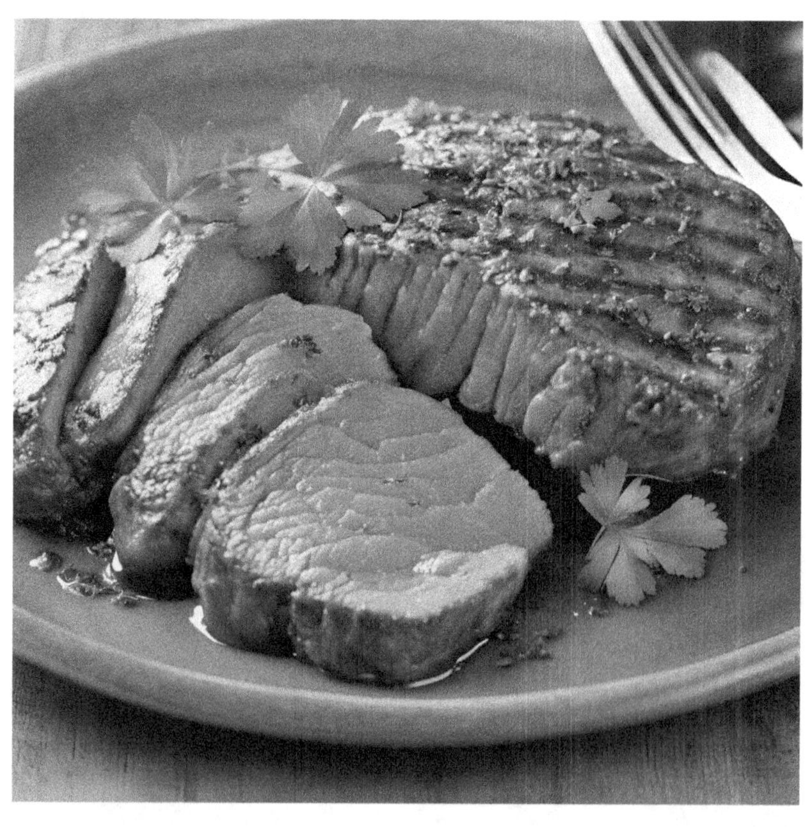

4. Chicken and Rice Casserole

Ingredients:

- 2 cups cooked rice
- 2 chicken breasts, cooked and shredded
- 1 cup frozen peas
- 1 cup diced carrots
- 1 cup low-sodium chicken broth
- 1/2 cup plain Greek yogurt
- 1 tsp dried thyme
- 1 tbsp olive oil

Instructions:

1. Preheat oven to 375°F (190°C).
2. In a large bowl, mix the cooked rice, shredded chicken, peas, and carrots.
3. Stir in chicken broth, Greek yogurt, and thyme until well combined.
4. Transfer the mixture to a greased baking dish and drizzle with olive oil.
5. Bake for 25-30 minutes, until bubbly and golden on top.

Nutrition Info Per Serving:

- Calories: 350
- Protein: 28g
- Carbohydrates: 40g
- Fat: 8g

Serves: 4

Cooking Time: 30 minutes

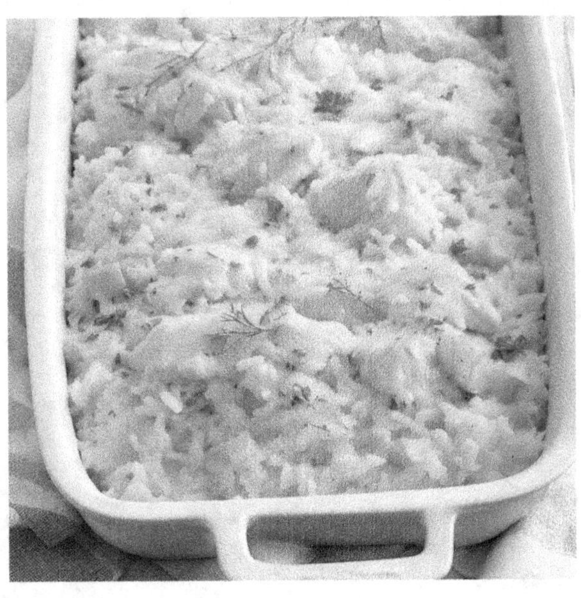

5. **Shrimp and Rice Pilaf**

Ingredients:

- 1 lb shrimp, peeled and deveined
- 1 cup rice
- 2 cups water
- 1/2 cup diced carrots
- 1/2 cup peas
- 1 tsp garlic powder
- 1 tbsp olive oil

Instructions:

1. In a large skillet, heat olive oil over medium heat.
2. Add rice and garlic powder, sauté for 2 minutes.
3. Add water, bring to a boil, then reduce heat to low.
4. Cover and simmer for 10 minutes.
5. Add shrimp, carrots, and peas. Cover and cook for an additional 10 minutes, until rice is tender and shrimp are cooked through.

Nutrition Info Per Serving:

- Calories: 340
- Protein: 25g
- Carbohydrates: 45g
- Fat: 7g

Serves: 4

Cooking Time: 25 minutes

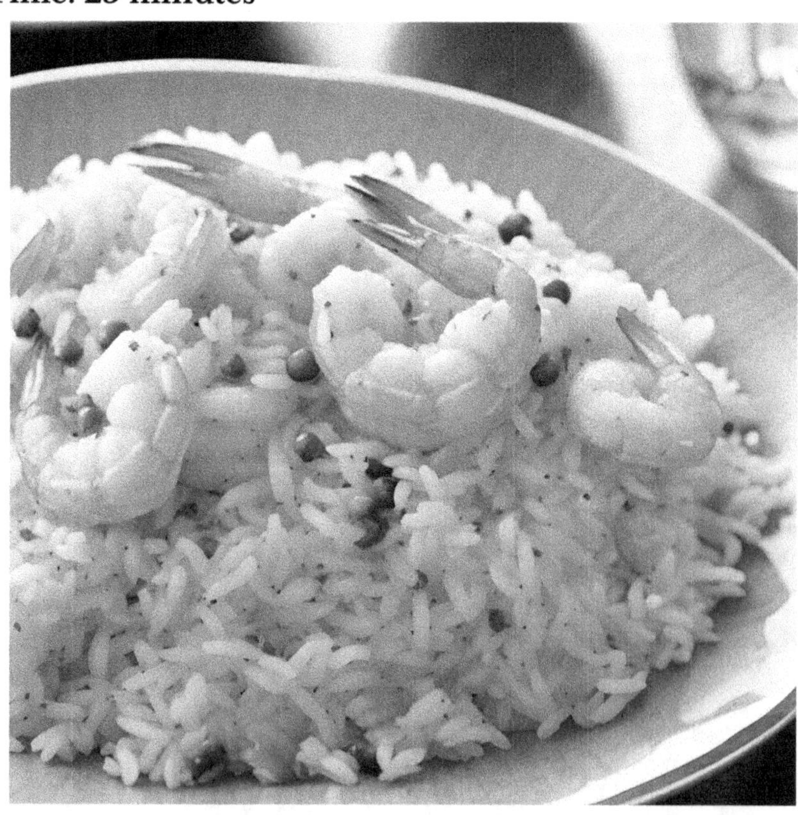

6. Lemon-Free Chicken Piccata

Ingredients:

- 4 chicken breasts, thinly sliced
- 1/2 cup flour
- 2 tbsp olive oil
- 1 cup low-sodium chicken broth
- 1 tbsp capers
- 1 tsp dried parsley

Instructions:

1. Dredge chicken breasts in flour.
2. Heat olive oil in a skillet over medium-high heat. Cook chicken until golden on each side, about 3-4 minutes per side.
3. Remove chicken from skillet. Add chicken broth and capers to the pan. Bring to a simmer.
4. Return chicken to the skillet, sprinkle with parsley, and cook for another 5 minutes.

Nutrition Info Per Serving:

- Calories: 290
- Protein: 27g
- Carbohydrates: 12g
- Fat: 14g

Serves: 4
Cooking Time: 20 minutes

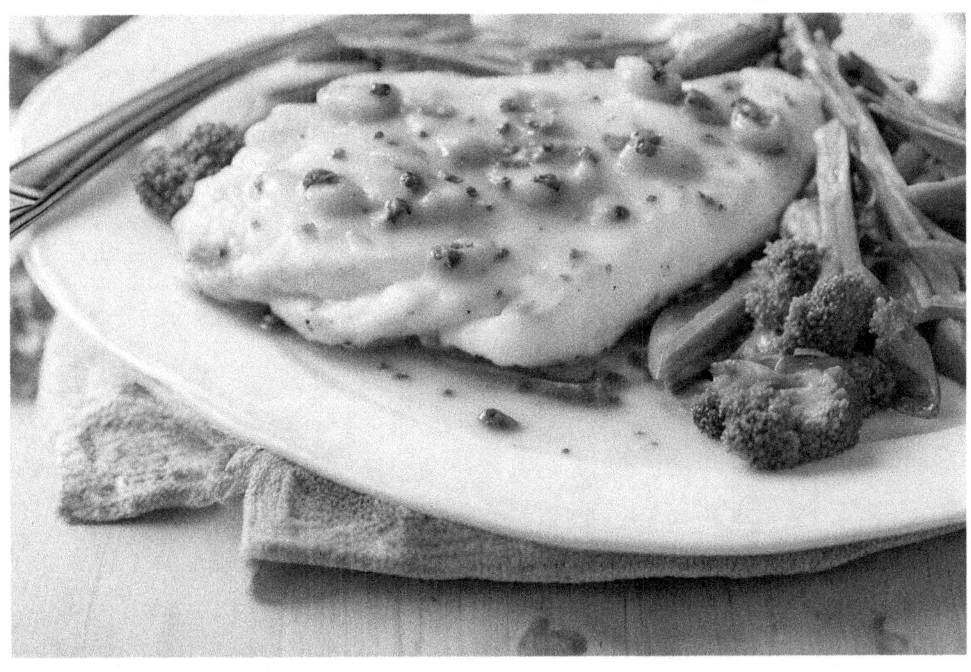

7. Garlic Butter Baked Cod

Ingredients:

- 4 cod fillets
- 4 tbsp butter, melted
- 2 tsp garlic powder
- 1 tbsp chopped fresh parsley
- 1 tbsp olive oil

Instructions:

1. Preheat oven to 400°F (200°C).
2. Place cod in a baking dish. Drizzle with olive oil and brush with melted butter mixed with garlic powder.
3. Bake for 12-15 minutes, until fish flakes easily with a fork.
4. Garnish with fresh parsley before serving.

Nutrition Info Per Serving:

- Calories: 230
- Protein: 22g
- Carbohydrates: 0g
- Fat: 15g

Serves: 4

Cooking Time: 15 minutes

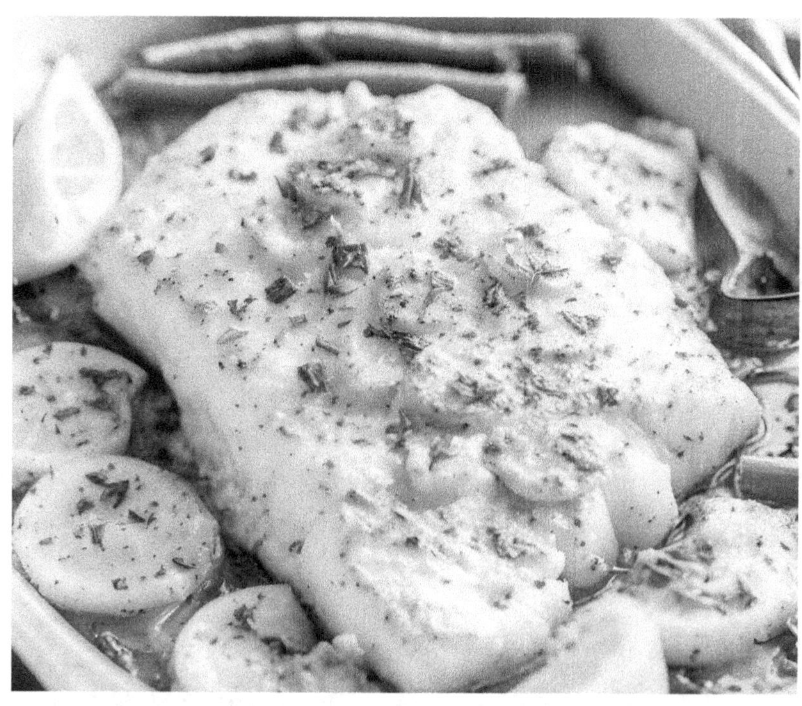

8. Pasta with Peas and Ham
Ingredients:

- 8 oz pasta
- 1 cup diced ham
- 1 cup frozen peas
- 1/2 cup cream
- 1 tbsp olive oil

Instructions:

1. Cook pasta according to package instructions.
2. In a skillet, heat olive oil over medium heat. Add ham and cook until lightly browned.
3. Add peas and cream to the skillet. Heat through.
4. Drain pasta and add to the skillet. Toss to combine.

Nutrition Info Per Serving:

- Calories: 400
- Protein: 17g
- Carbohydrates: 52g
- Fat: 14g

Serves: 4
Cooking Time: 20 minutes

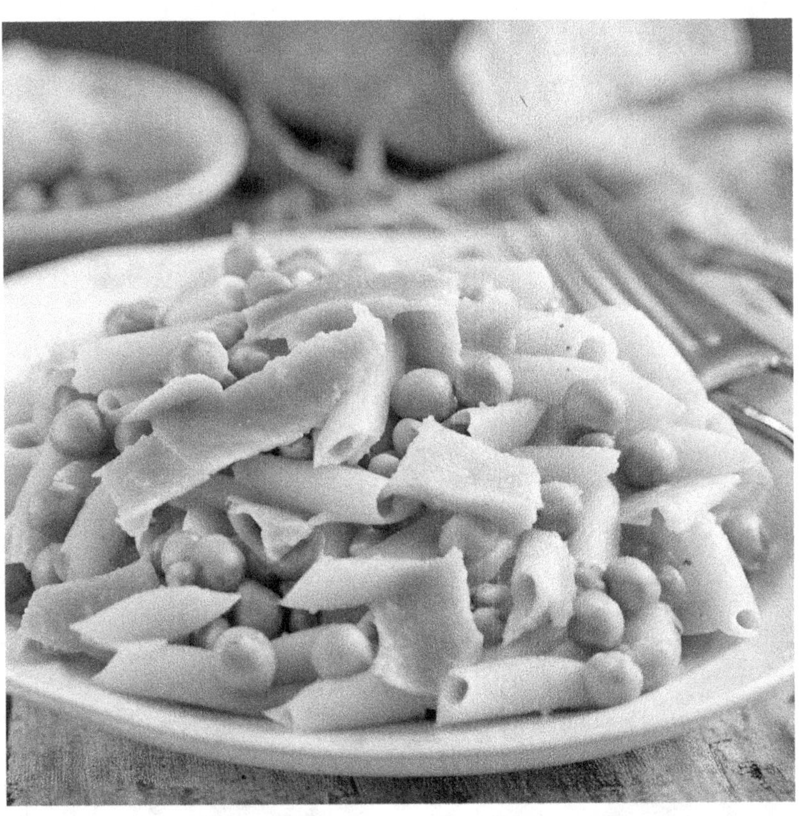

9. Mushroom Risotto

Ingredients:

- 1 cup Arborio rice
- 1/2 lb mushrooms, sliced
- 4 cups vegetable broth
- 1/2 cup Parmesan cheese, grated
- 1 tbsp olive oil
- 1 tsp thyme

Instructions:

1. In a large pan, heat olive oil over medium heat. Add mushrooms and cook until soft.
2. Add rice and stir for 1 minute.
3. Gradually add broth, 1 cup at a time, stirring constantly until each addition is absorbed before adding the next.
4. Once all broth is absorbed and rice is creamy, stir in Parmesan and thyme.

Nutrition Info Per Serving:

- Calories: 350
- Protein: 12g
- Carbohydrates: 55g
- Fat: 9g

Serves: 4

Cooking Time: 40 minutes

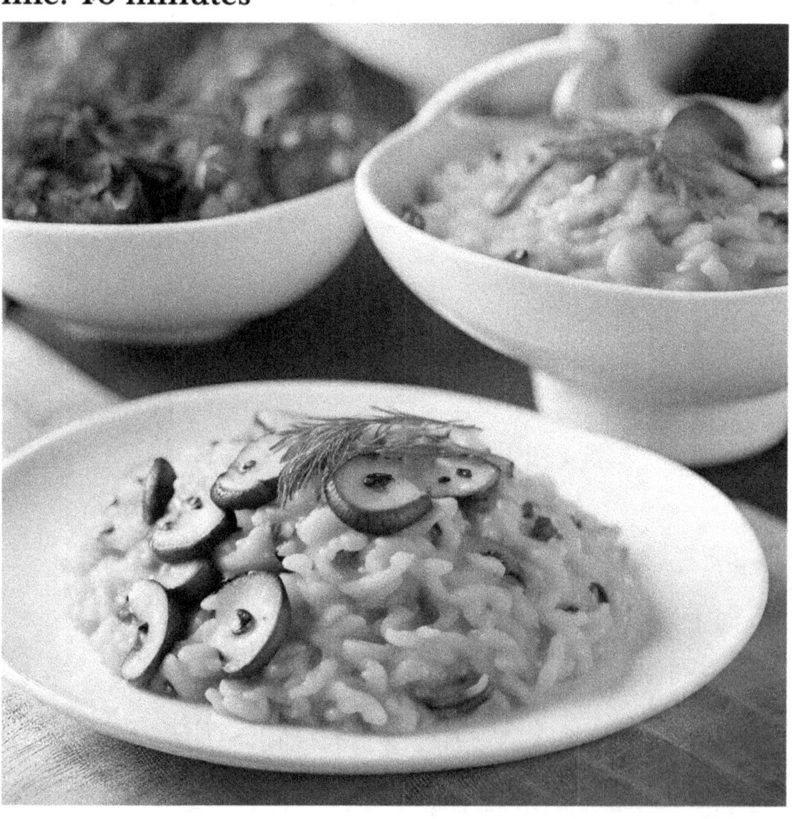

10. Vegetarian Chili

Ingredients:

- 1 cup chopped onions
- 1 cup chopped bell peppers
- 1 cup diced carrots
- 1 cup corn kernels
- 1 can (15 oz) black beans, drained and rinsed
- 1 can (15 oz) kidney beans, drained and rinsed
- 2 cups vegetable broth
- 1 tbsp chili powder
- 1 tbsp cumin
- 1 tbsp olive oil

Instructions:

1. In a large pot, heat olive oil over medium heat. Add onions, bell peppers, and carrots. Cook until soft.
2. Add beans, corn, broth, chili powder, and cumin. Bring to a boil.
3. Reduce heat and simmer for 30 minutes, stirring occasionally.

Nutrition Info Per Serving:

- Calories: 250
- Protein: 14g
- Carbohydrates: 45g
- Fat: 4g

Serves: 6
Cooking Time: 40 minutes

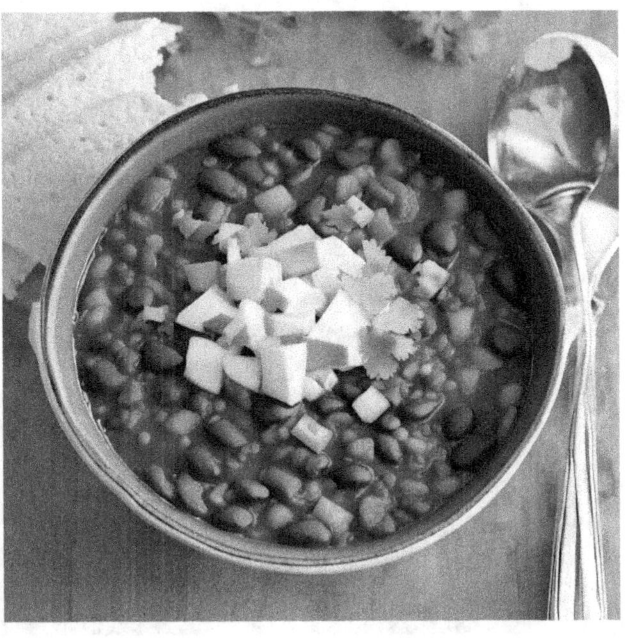

11. Grilled Lamb Chops with Mint

Ingredients:

- 8 lamb chops
- 2 tbsp olive oil
- 1/4 cup fresh mint, finely chopped
- 2 cloves garlic, minced
- 1 tbsp honey

Instructions:

1. Mix olive oil, mint, garlic, and honey in a bowl.
2. Marinate lamb chops in the mixture for at least 1 hour in the refrigerator.
3. Preheat grill to medium-high heat.
4. Grill lamb chops for about 4-5 minutes on each side or until desired doneness.

Nutrition Info Per Serving:

- Calories: 350
- Protein: 24g
- Carbohydrates: 5g
- Fat: 26g

Serves: 4Cooking Time: 10 minutes plus marinating

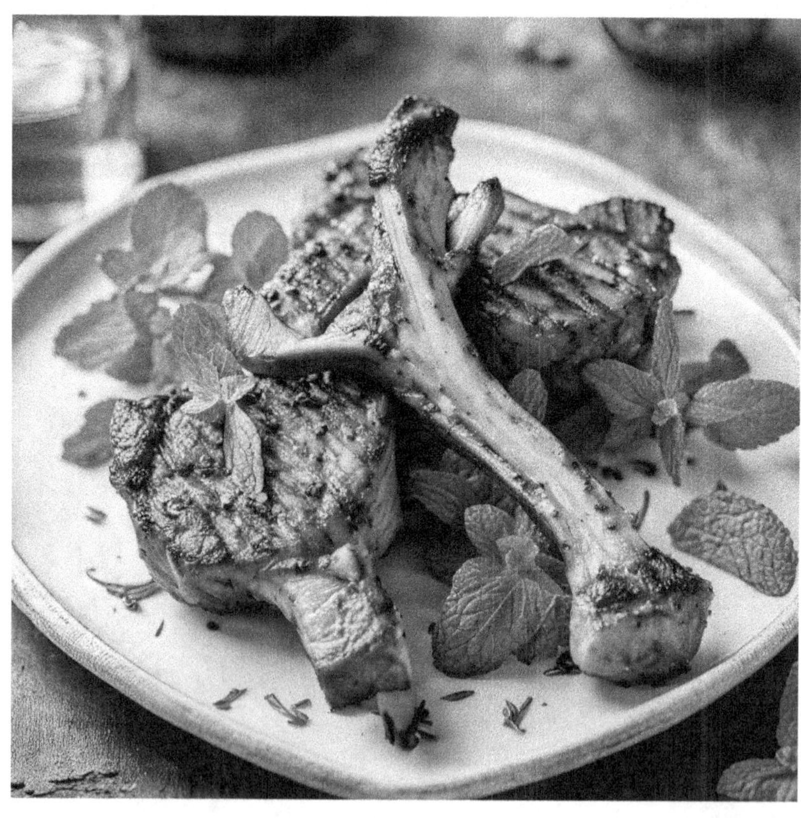

12. Herbed Baked Pollock

Ingredients:

- 4 pollock fillets
- 2 tbsp olive oil
- 1 tsp dried dill
- 1 tsp dried parsley
- 1 lemon, sliced (for garnish)

Instructions:

1. Preheat oven to 375°F (190°C).
2. Place pollock fillets in a baking dish and drizzle with olive oil.
3. Sprinkle with dill and parsley.
4. Bake for 20 minutes or until fish flakes easily with a fork.
5. Garnish with lemon slices.

Nutrition Info Per Serving:

- Calories: 200
- Protein: 23g
- Carbohydrates: 1g
- Fat: 12g

Serves: 4
Cooking Time: 20 minutes

13. Chicken Alfredo Pasta

Ingredients:

- 8 oz fettuccine
- 2 chicken breasts, cooked and sliced
- 1 cup cream
- 1/2 cup grated Parmesan cheese
- 1 tbsp olive oil
- 1 tsp dried basil

Instructions:

1. Cook fettuccine according to package instructions.
2. In a pan, heat olive oil over medium heat. Add sliced chicken and basil, cook until heated through.
3. Lower heat and add cream and Parmesan cheese, stirring until sauce thickens.
4. Toss cooked pasta with the sauce and chicken.

Nutrition Info Per Serving:

- Calories: 530
- Protein: 32g
- Carbohydrates: 44g
- Fat: 26g

Serves: 4

Cooking Time: 20 minutes

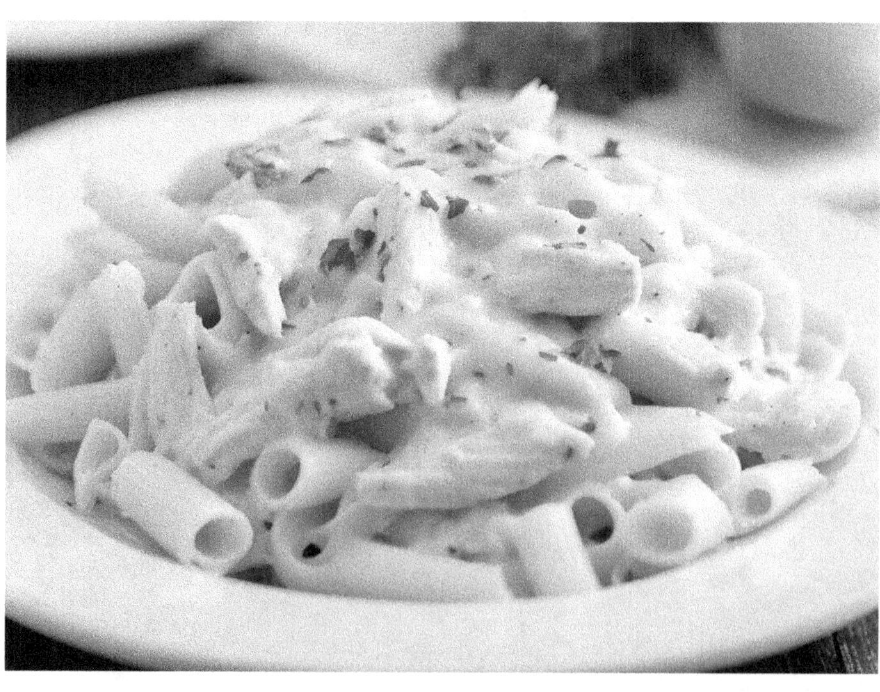

14. Roasted Duck with Wild Rice

Ingredients:

- 1 whole duck
- 2 cups wild rice
- 4 cups water
- 1 tbsp olive oil
- 1 tsp dried thyme

Instructions:

1. Preheat oven to 350°F (175°C).
2. Rinse duck and pat dry. Rub with olive oil and thyme.
3. Roast in the oven for about 1.5 hours or until the internal temperature reaches 165°F (74°C).
4. Cook wild rice in water as per package instructions.

Nutrition Info Per Serving:

- Calories: 600
- Protein: 45g
- Carbohydrates: 45g
- Fat: 25g

Serves: 4

Cooking Time: 90 minutes

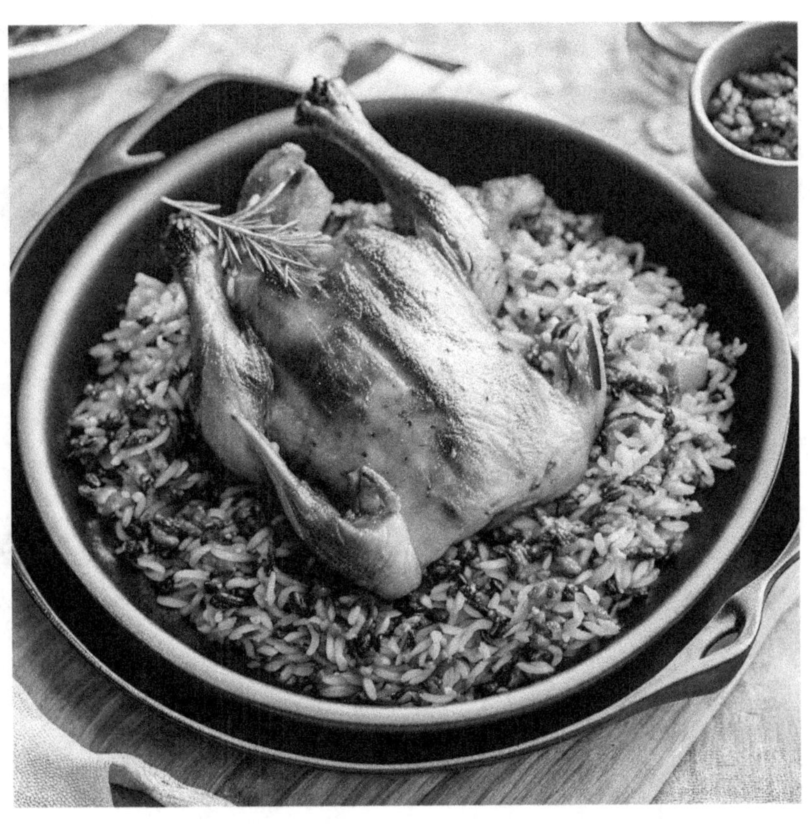

15. Rabbit Stew with Vegetables

Ingredients:

- 1 rabbit, cut into pieces
- 4 cups water
- 1 cup diced carrots
- 1 cup diced celery
- 1 cup diced potatoes
- 1 tbsp olive oil
- 1 tsp dried rosemary

Instructions:

1. In a large pot, heat olive oil over medium heat. Brown rabbit pieces on all sides.
2. Add water, carrots, celery, potatoes, and rosemary.
3. Bring to a boil, then reduce heat and simmer for 1 hour or until rabbit is tender.

Nutrition Info Per Serving:

- Calories: 310
- Protein: 25g
- Carbohydrates: 23g
- Fat: 14g

Serves: 4Cooking Time: 70 minutes

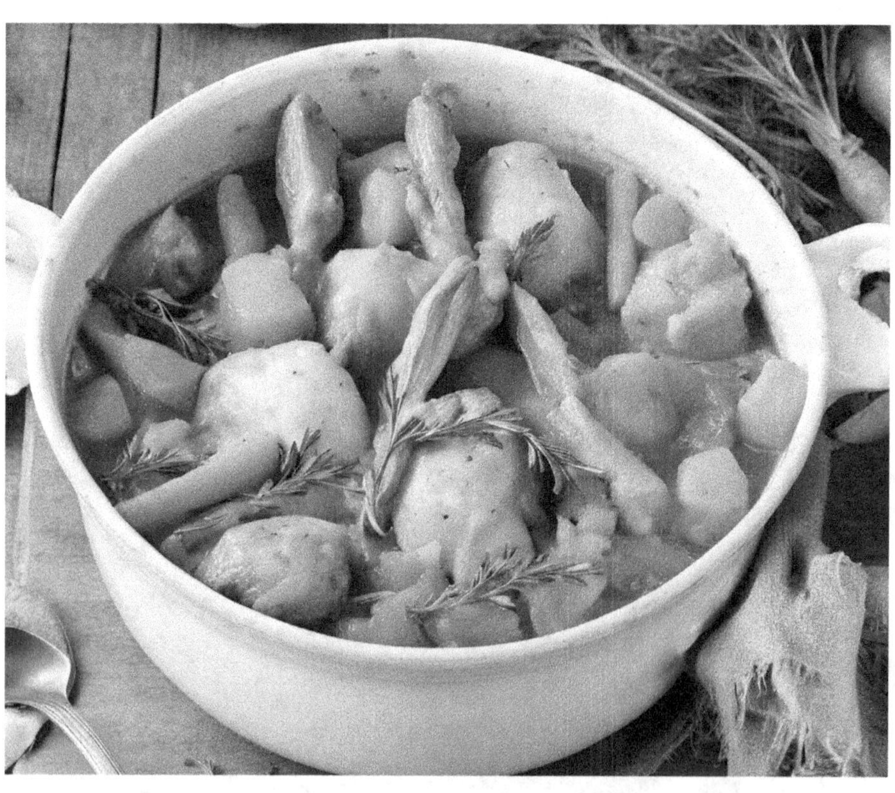

16. Squash and Carrot Casserole

Ingredients:

- 2 cups sliced squash
- 2 cups sliced carrots
- 1/2 cup cream
- 1/2 cup grated cheddar cheese
- 1 tbsp olive oil

Instructions:

1. Preheat oven to 350°F (175°C).
2. In a casserole dish, layer the sliced squash and carrots. Drizzle with olive oil.
3. Pour cream evenly over the vegetables.
4. Sprinkle with grated cheddar cheese.
5. Bake in the preheated oven for 30 minutes, until vegetables are tender and the top is golden brown.

Nutrition Info Per Serving:

- Calories: 280
- Protein: 7g
- Carbohydrates: 18g
- Fat: 21g

Serves: 4
Cooking Time: 30 minutes

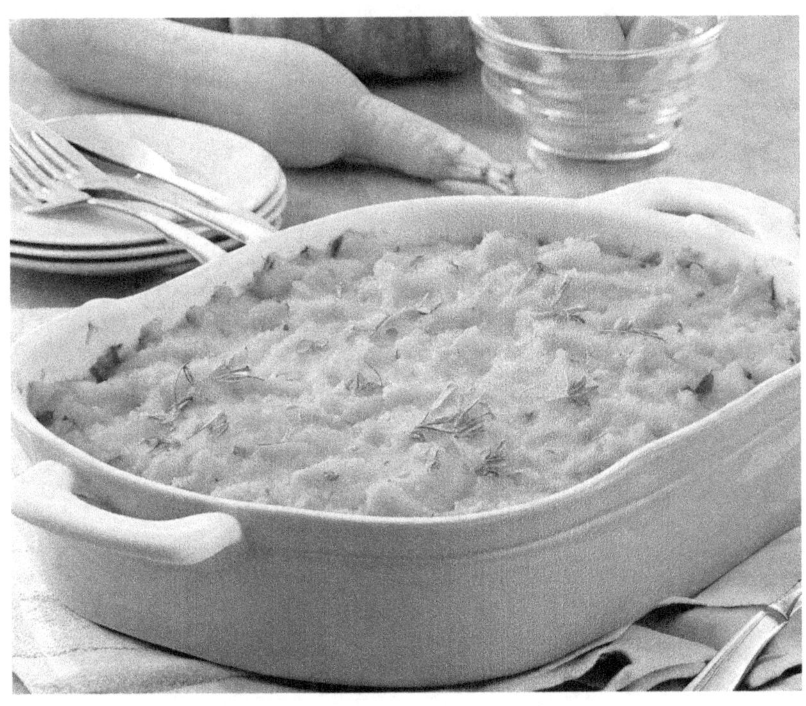

17. Flounder with Parsley Sauce

Ingredients:

- 4 flounder fillets
- 2 tbsp butter
- 1/4 cup chopped fresh parsley
- 1 cup milk
- 1 tbsp flour

Instructions:

1. Preheat the oven to 375°F (190°C).
2. Place flounder fillets in a baking dish.
3. In a small saucepan, melt butter over medium heat, stir in flour to make a roux.
4. Gradually add milk, stirring continuously until the sauce thickens.
5. Stir in chopped parsley and pour the sauce over the flounder.
6. Bake for 20 minutes, until the fish is flaky.

Nutrition Info Per Serving:

- Calories: 220
- Protein: 21g
- Carbohydrates: 6g
- Fat: 12g

Serves: 4
Cooking Time: 25 minutes

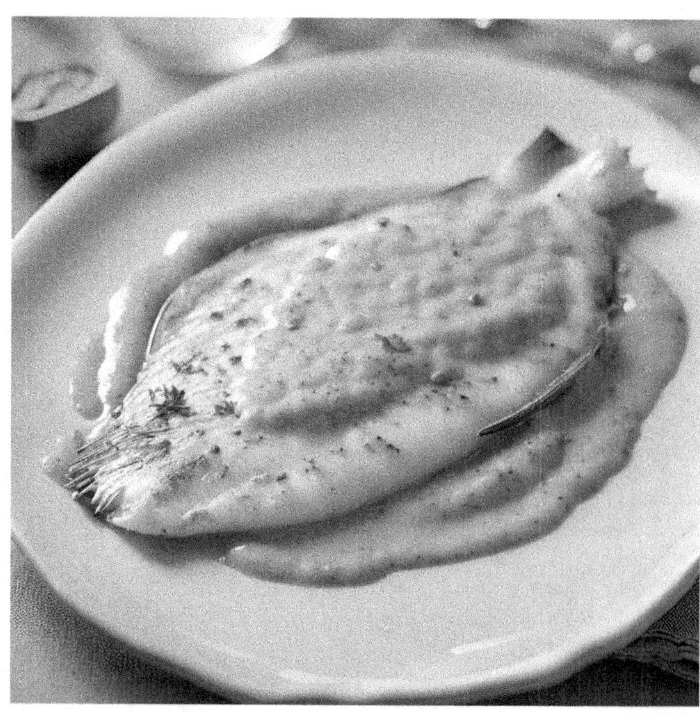

18. Cauliflower Steak with Herbs

Ingredients:

- 4 large cauliflower slices (steaks)
- 2 tbsp olive oil
- 1 tsp dried herbs (thyme, rosemary)
- 1 tbsp lemon zest (optional for garnish)

Instructions:

1. Preheat the oven to 400°F (200°C).
2. Brush cauliflower steaks with olive oil and sprinkle with dried herbs.
3. Bake for 25 minutes, until tender and edges are crispy.
4. Garnish with lemon zest if using.

Nutrition Info Per Serving:

- Calories: 140
- Protein: 4g
- Carbohydrates: 10g
- Fat: 10g

Serves: 4

Cooking Time: 25 minutes

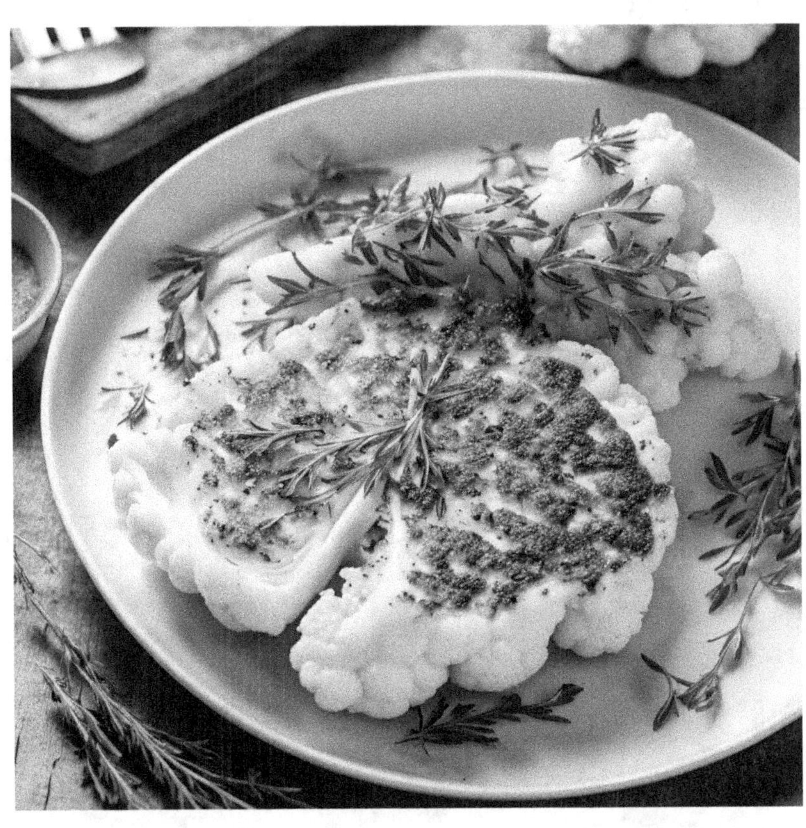

19. Venison Stew

Ingredients:

- 2 lbs venison, cubed
- 4 cups beef broth
- 1 cup diced potatoes
- 1 cup sliced carrots
- 1 cup diced onions
- 1 tbsp olive oil
- 1 tsp dried thyme

Instructions:

1. In a large pot, heat olive oil over medium heat. Brown the venison cubes.
2. Add onions and sauté until translucent.
3. Add beef broth, potatoes, carrots, and thyme.
4. Bring to a boil, then reduce heat and simmer for 2 hours, until meat is tender.

Nutrition Info Per Serving:

- Calories: 350
- Protein: 35g
- Carbohydrates: 15g
- Fat: 15g

Serves: 4

Cooking Time: 130 minutes

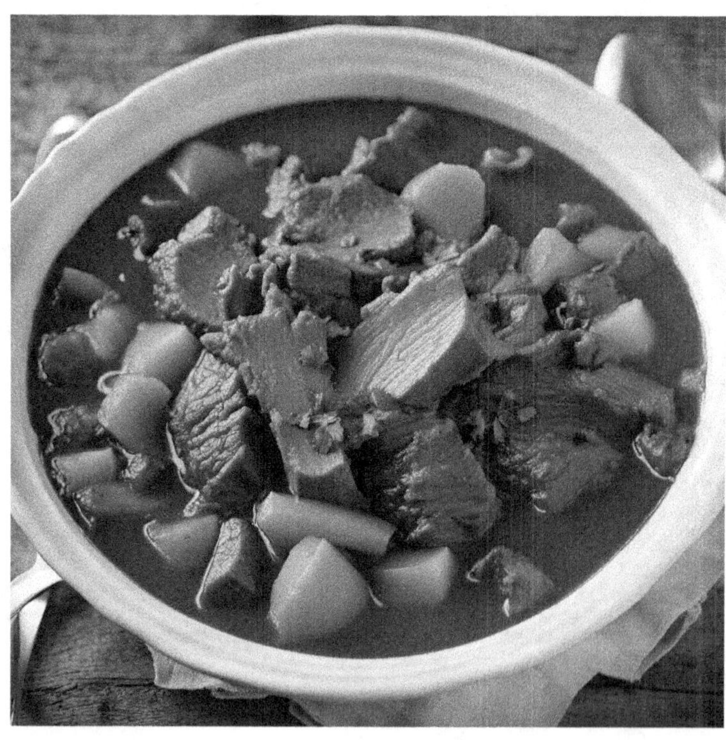

20. Herb-Roasted Quail

Ingredients:

- 8 quail
- 2 tbsp olive oil

1 tsp dried rosemary

- 1 tsp dried thyme
- 1 tsp garlic powder

Instructions:

1. Preheat oven to 400°F (200°C).
2. Rub each quail with olive oil and then sprinkle evenly with rosemary, thyme, and garlic powder.
3. Place quail in a roasting pan and roast for about 25 minutes, until fully cooked and golden.

Nutrition Info Per Serving:

- Calories: 310
- Protein: 24g
- Carbohydrates: 0g
- Fat: 23g

Serves: 4Cooking Time: 25 minutes

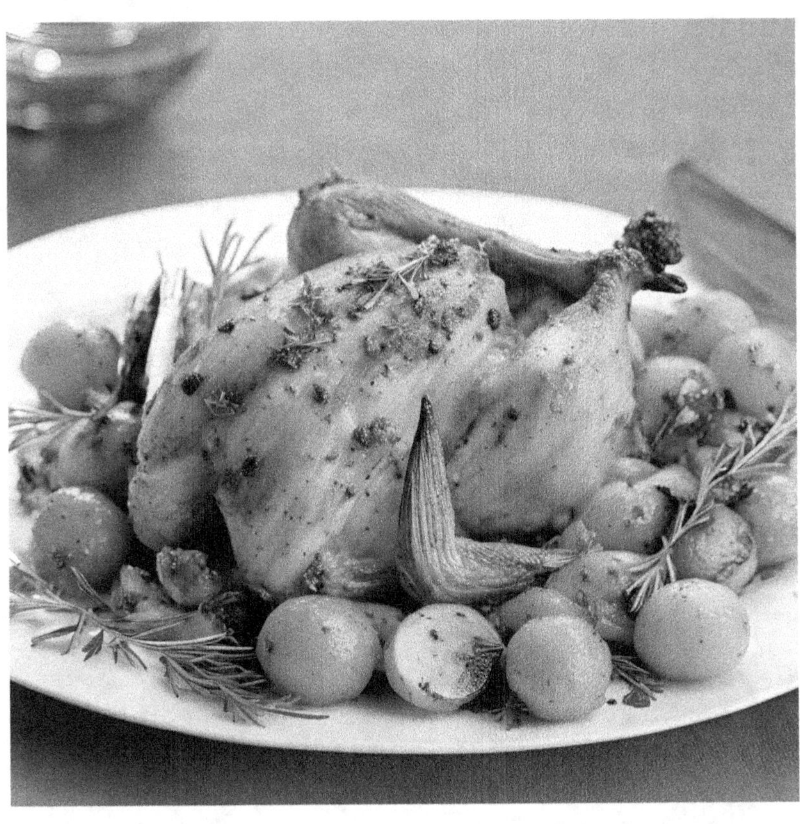

Soups and Salad Recipes

1. Asparagus Cream Soup

Ingredients:

- 1 lb asparagus, trimmed and chopped
- 1 onion, chopped
- 2 cups vegetable broth
- 1 cup cream
- 1 tbsp olive oil
- 1 tsp garlic powder

Instructions:

1. In a large pot, heat olive oil over medium heat. Sauté onions until translucent.
2. Add asparagus and garlic powder, cook for 5 minutes.
3. Pour in vegetable broth and bring to a boil. Reduce heat and simmer for 15 minutes.
4. Blend the mixture until smooth, then stir in cream and heat through.

Nutrition Info Per Serving:

- Calories: 220
- Protein: 4g
- Carbohydrates: 12g
- Fat: 18g

Serves: 4

Cooking Time: 30 minutes

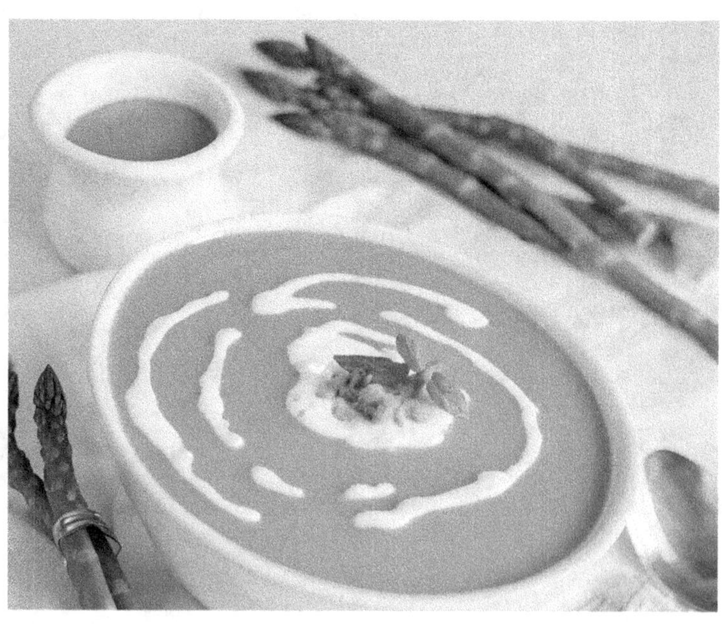

2. Barley and Mushroom Soup

Ingredients:

- 1 cup pearl barley, rinsed
- 1 lb mushrooms, sliced
- 6 cups vegetable broth
- 1 onion, chopped
- 1 tbsp olive oil
- 1 tsp dried thyme

Instructions:

1. In a large pot, heat olive oil over medium heat. Sauté onions until translucent.
2. Add mushrooms and thyme, cook until mushrooms are soft.
3. Add barley and vegetable broth. Bring to a boil, then reduce heat and simmer for 40 minutes, or until barley is tender.

Nutrition Info Per Serving:

- Calories: 180
- Protein: 6g
- Carbohydrates: 32g
- Fat: 4g

Serves: 4Cooking Time: 50 minutes

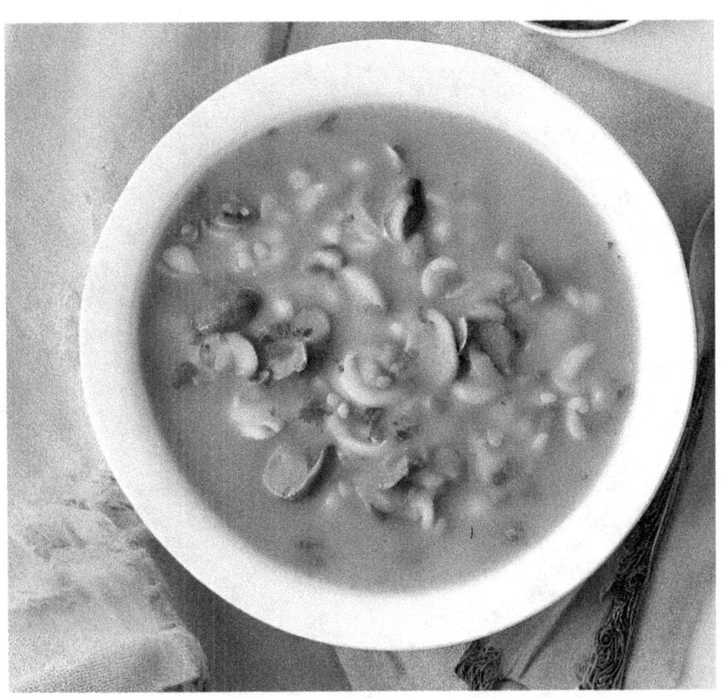

3. Broccoli Cheese Soup

Ingredients:

- 2 cups chopped broccoli
- 2 cups vegetable broth
- 1 cup cheddar cheese, grated
- 1 cup cream
- 1 onion, chopped
- 1 tbsp olive oil
- 1 tsp garlic powder

Instructions:

1. In a pot, heat olive oil over medium heat. Sauté onion until translucent.
2. Add broccoli, garlic powder, and vegetable broth. Cook until broccoli is tender, about 10 minutes.
3. Blend the mixture until smooth. Return to the pot, stir in cream and cheese until melted and combined.

Nutrition Info Per Serving:

- Calories: 350
- Protein: 15g
- Carbohydrates: 15g
- Fat: 25g

Serves: 4

Cooking Time: 25 minutes

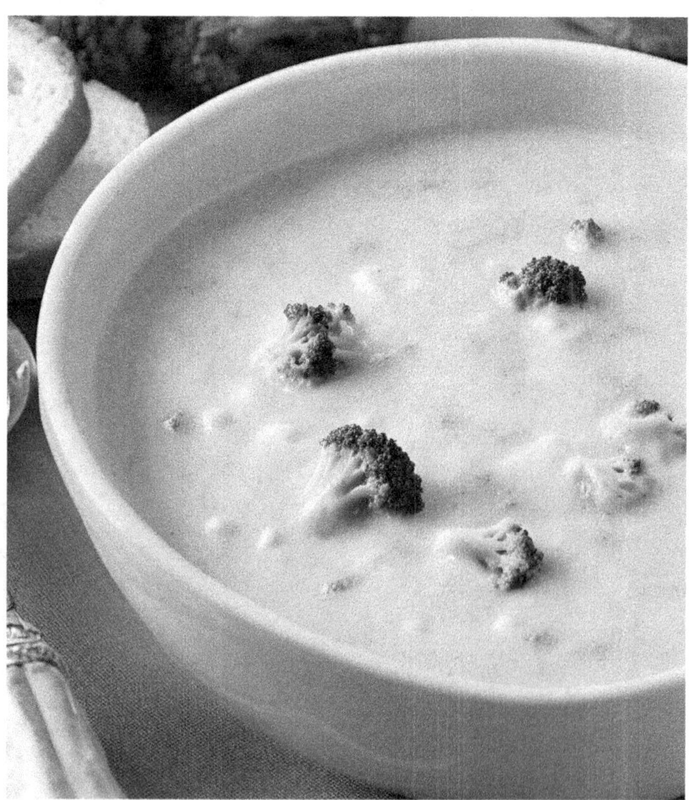

4. Chicken Noodle Soup

Ingredients:

- 2 chicken breasts, cooked and shredded
- 6 cups chicken broth
- 2 cups egg noodles
- 1 cup sliced carrots
- 1 cup sliced celery
- 1 onion, chopped
- 1 tbsp olive oil
- 1 tsp dried parsley

Instructions:

1. In a large pot, heat olive oil over medium heat. Sauté onions, carrots, and celery until soft.
2. Add chicken broth and bring to a boil.
3. Add egg noodles and cook for 10 minutes, or until tender.
4. Stir in shredded chicken and parsley, and heat through.

Nutrition Info Per Serving:

- Calories: 250
- Protein: 20g
- Carbohydrates: 25g
- Fat: 7g

Serves: 4
Cooking Time: 30 minutes

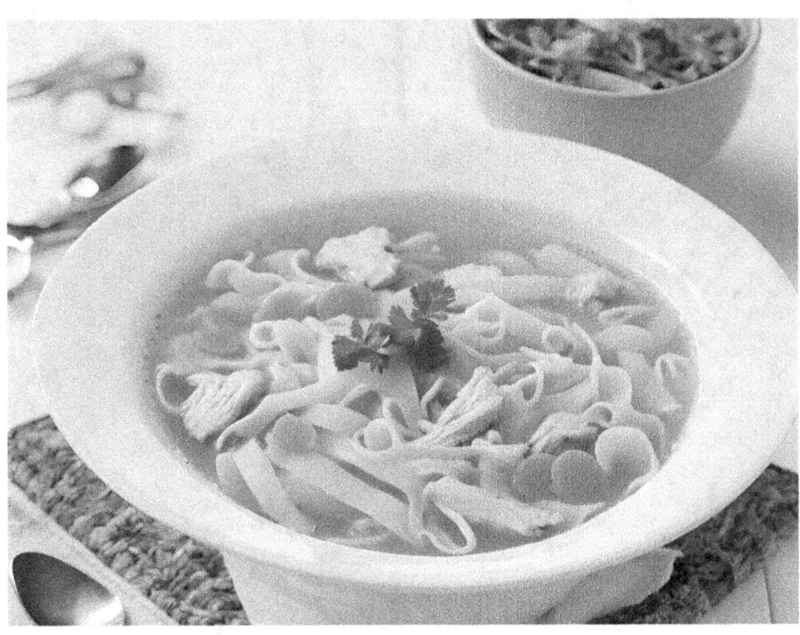

5. Corn Chowder

Ingredients:

- 2 cups corn kernels
- 2 cups vegetable broth
- 1 cup diced potatoes
- 1 cup cream
- 1 onion, chopped
- 1 tbsp olive oil
- 1 tsp dried thyme

Instructions:

1. In a pot, heat olive oil over medium heat. Sauté onion until translucent.
2. Add potatoes, corn, thyme, and vegetable broth. Bring to a boil, then reduce heat and simmer for 20 minutes, until potatoes are tender.
3. Blend half of the soup for a creamy texture, then return to the pot. Stir in cream and heat through.

Nutrition Info Per Serving:

- Calories: 280
- Protein: 5g
- Carbohydrates: 35g
- Fat: 14g

Serves: 4
Cooking Time: 35 minutes

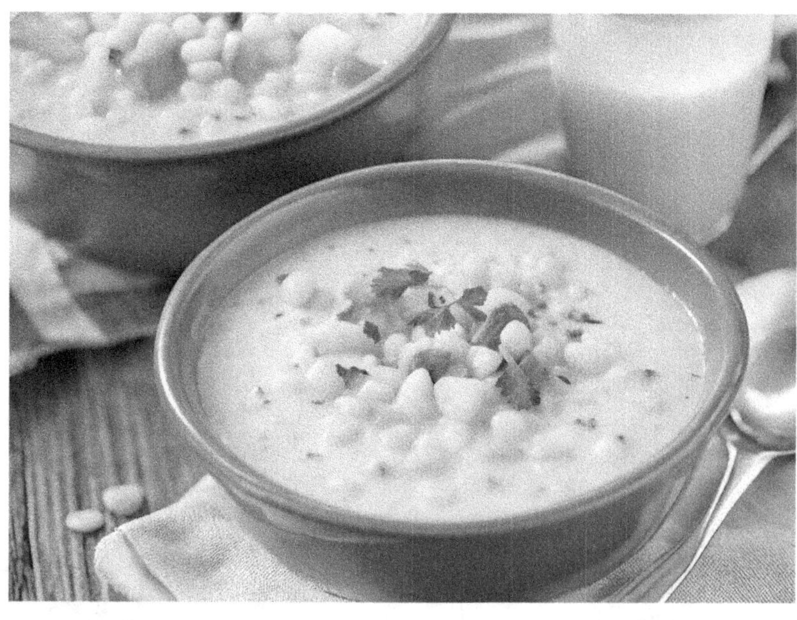

6. Egg Drop Soup

Ingredients:

- 4 cups chicken broth
- 2 eggs, beaten
- 1 tbsp cornstarch mixed with 2 tbsp water
- 1 tsp sesame oil
- 1 tbsp chopped green onions

Instructions:

1. Bring chicken broth to a boil in a pot.
2. Slowly pour in the beaten eggs while stirring the broth gently.
3. Add cornstarch mixture to thicken the soup.
4. Drizzle with sesame oil and garnish with green onions before serving.

Nutrition Info Per Serving:

- Calories: 90
- Protein: 6g
- Carbohydrates: 4g
- Fat: 5g

Serves: 4

Cooking Time: 15 minutes

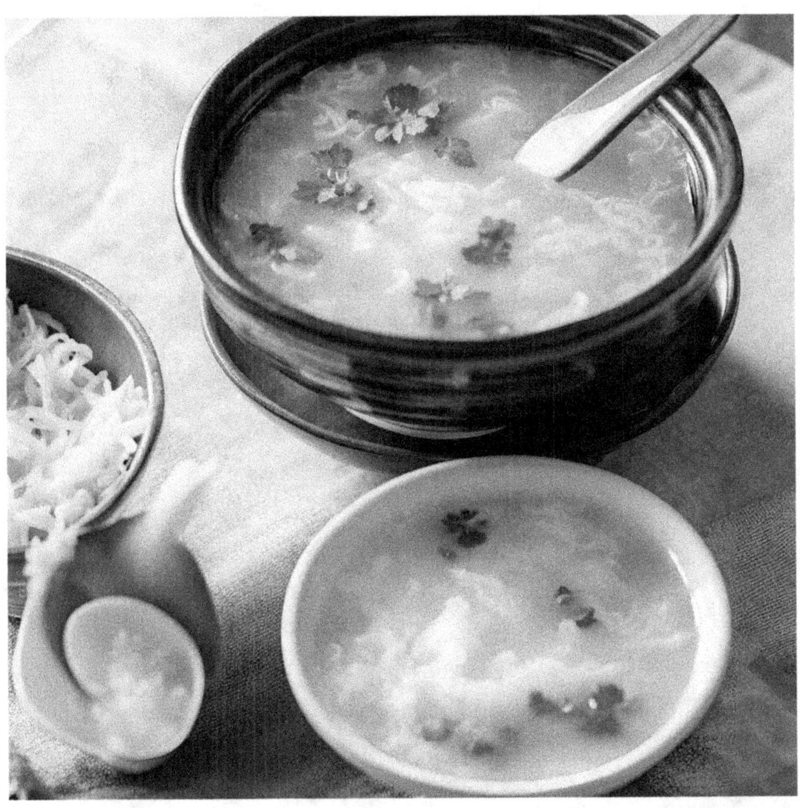

7. Apple Walnut Salad

Ingredients:

- 2 apples, cored and chopped
- 1/2 cup walnuts, chopped
- 1/2 cup celery, sliced
- 1/4 cup mayonnaise
- 1/4 cup plain yogurt

Instructions:

1. In a large bowl, combine apples, walnuts, and celery.
2. Mix mayonnaise and yogurt, then toss with the apple mixture until well coated.

Nutrition Info Per Serving:

- Calories: 250
- Protein: 4g
- Carbohydrates: 20g
- Fat: 18g

Serves: 4
Cooking Time: 10 minutes

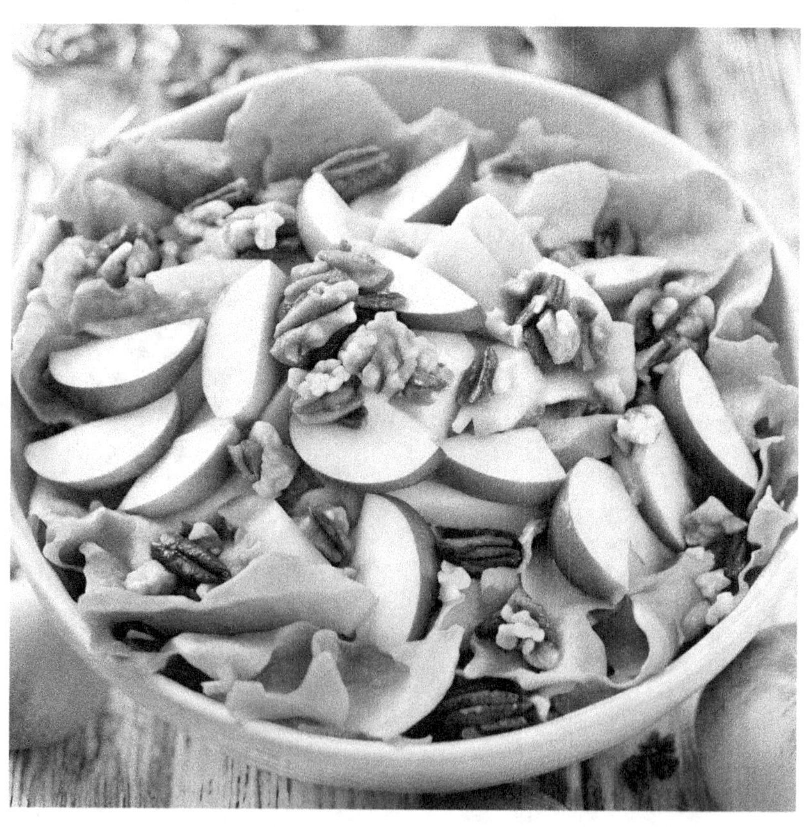

8. Chicken and Avocado Salad

Ingredients:

- 2 chicken breasts, cooked and shredded
- 2 avocados, peeled and diced
- 1/2 cup diced cucumber
- 1/4 cup plain yogurt
- 1 tbsp olive oil
- 1 tsp dried dill

Instructions:

1. In a large bowl, combine shredded chicken, avocados, and cucumber.
2. Mix yogurt, olive oil, and dill in a small bowl, then pour over the chicken mixture and toss to coat.

Nutrition Info Per Serving:

- Calories: 320
- Protein: 25g
- Carbohydrates: 12g
- Fat: 20g

Serves: 4
Cooking Time: 10 minutes

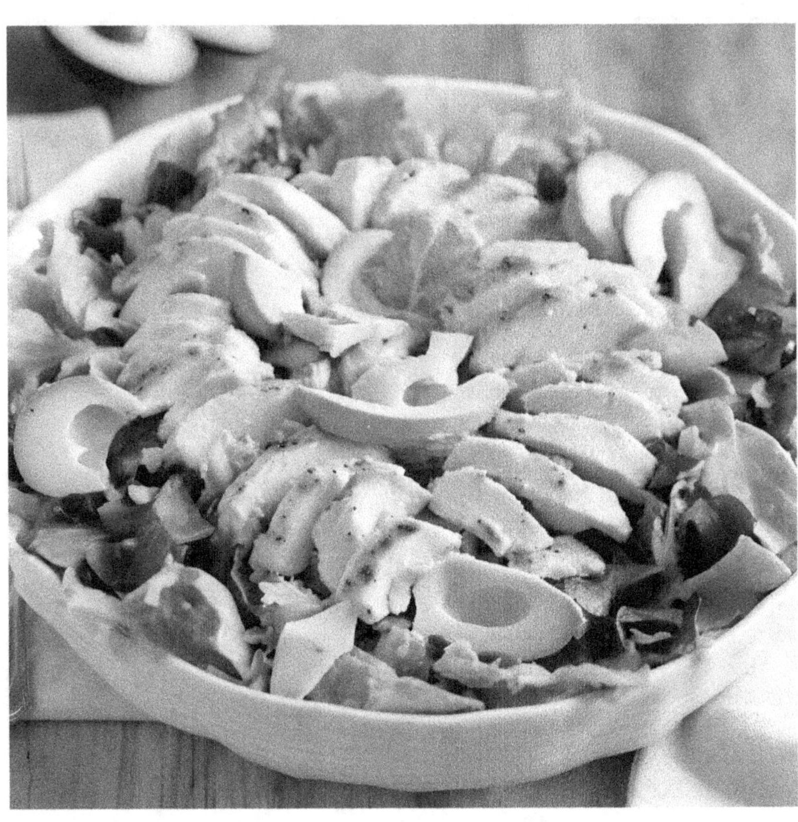

9. Carrot and Raisin Salad
Ingredients:

- 2 cups grated carrots
- 1/2 cup raisins
- 1/4 cup plain yogurt
- 1 tbsp honey
- 1/2 tsp cinnamon

Instructions:

1. In a large bowl, combine grated carrots and raisins.
2. Mix yogurt, honey, and cinnamon in a small bowl, then pour over the carrot mixture and toss to coat evenly.

Nutrition Info Per Serving:

- Calories: 140
- Protein: 2g
- Carbohydrates: 32g
- Fat: 1g

Serves: 4
Cooking Time: 10 minutes

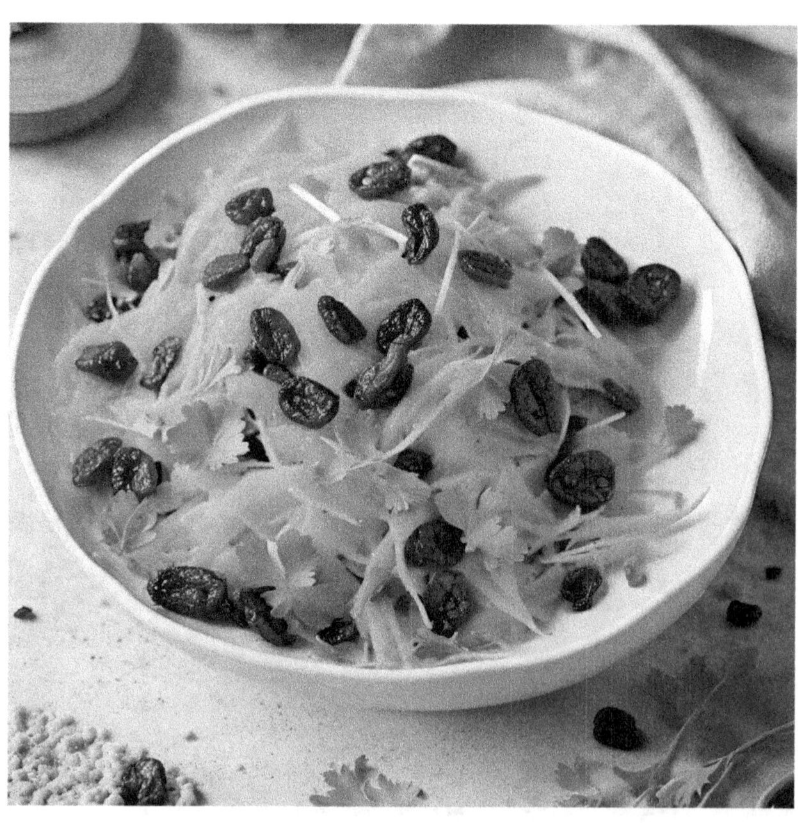

10. Green Bean Soup

Ingredients:

- 2 cups green beans, trimmed and chopped
- 4 cups vegetable broth
- 1 onion, chopped
- 1 tbsp olive oil
- 1 tsp dried dill

Instructions:

1. In a pot, heat olive oil over medium heat. Sauté onion until translucent.
2. Add green beans and vegetable broth. Bring to a boil, then simmer for 20 minutes until beans are tender.
3. Puree soup in a blender until smooth, then return to the pot and reheat. Stir in dill before serving.

Nutrition Info Per Serving:

- Calories: 80
- Protein: 2g
- Carbohydrates: 12g
- Fat: 3g

Serves: 4

Cooking Time: 30 minutes

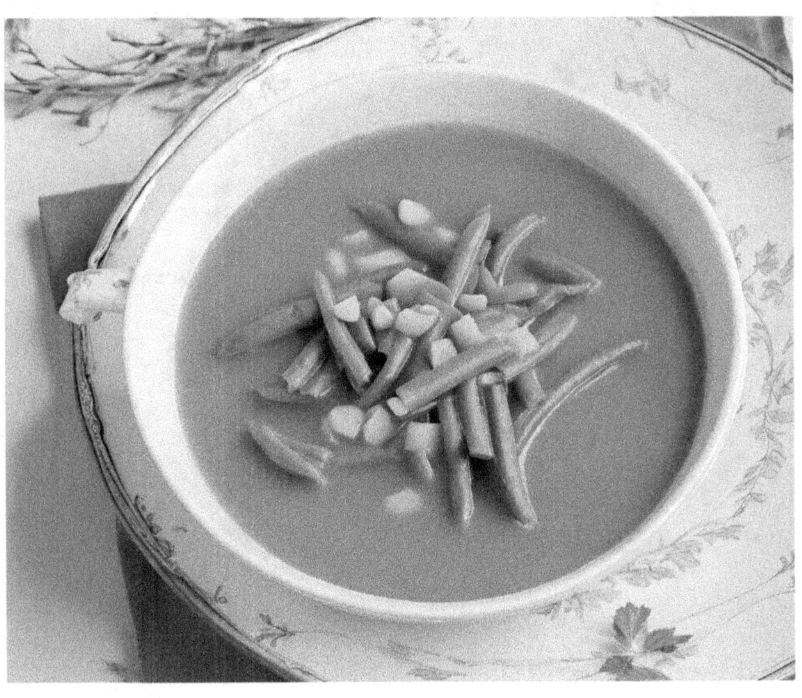

11. Leek and Potato Soup

Ingredients:

- 3 leeks, cleaned and sliced
- 2 potatoes, peeled and diced
- 4 cups vegetable broth
- 1 tbsp olive oil
- 1 tsp thyme

Instructions:

1. In a large pot, heat olive oil over medium heat. Add leeks and sauté until softened.
2. Add potatoes and vegetable broth. Bring to a boil, then reduce heat and simmer for 25 minutes until potatoes are soft.
3. Puree the soup until smooth, then reheat and stir in thyme.

Nutrition Info Per Serving:

- Calories: 200
- Protein: 4g
- Carbohydrates: 38g
- Fat: 4g

Serves: 4

Cooking Time: 35 minutes

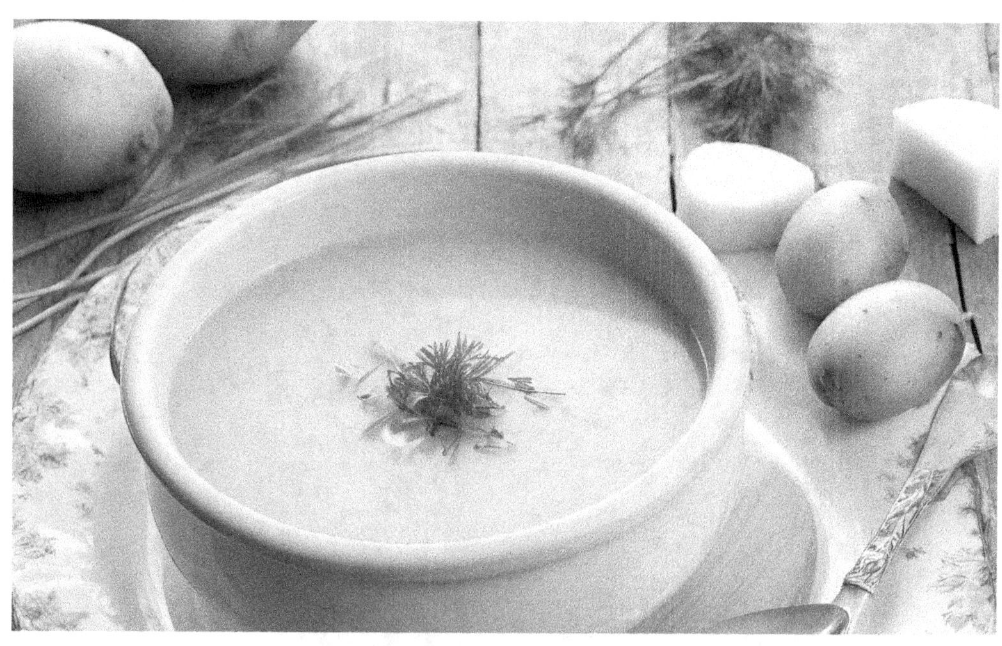

12. Oatmeal Soup

Ingredients:

- 1 cup rolled oats
- 4 cups vegetable broth
- 1 onion, chopped
- 1 carrot, chopped
- 1 tbsp olive oil
- 1 tsp dried parsley

Instructions:

1. In a pot, heat olive oil over medium heat. Sauté onion and carrot until softened.
2. Add oats and vegetable broth. Bring to a boil, then reduce heat and simmer for 15 minutes until oats are cooked.
3. Stir in parsley before serving.

Nutrition Info Per Serving:

- Calories: 180
- Protein: 6g
- Carbohydrates: 30g
- Fat: 5g

Serves: 4

Cooking Time: 25 minutes

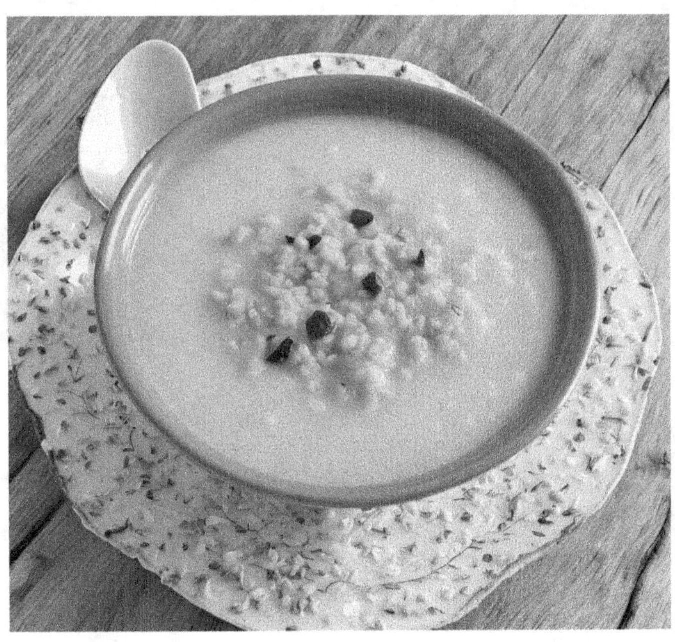

13. Rice and Almond Soup

Ingredients:

- 1 cup cooked rice
- 4 cups almond milk
- 1/4 cup slivered almonds
- 1 tbsp honey
- 1 tsp cinnamon

Instructions:

1. In a pot, combine cooked rice, almond milk, slivered almonds, honey, and cinnamon.
2. Heat over medium heat until warm, stirring occasionally.

Nutrition Info Per Serving:

- Calories: 220
- Protein: 5g
- Carbohydrates: 35g
- Fat: 7g

Serves: 4

Cooking Time: 15 minutes

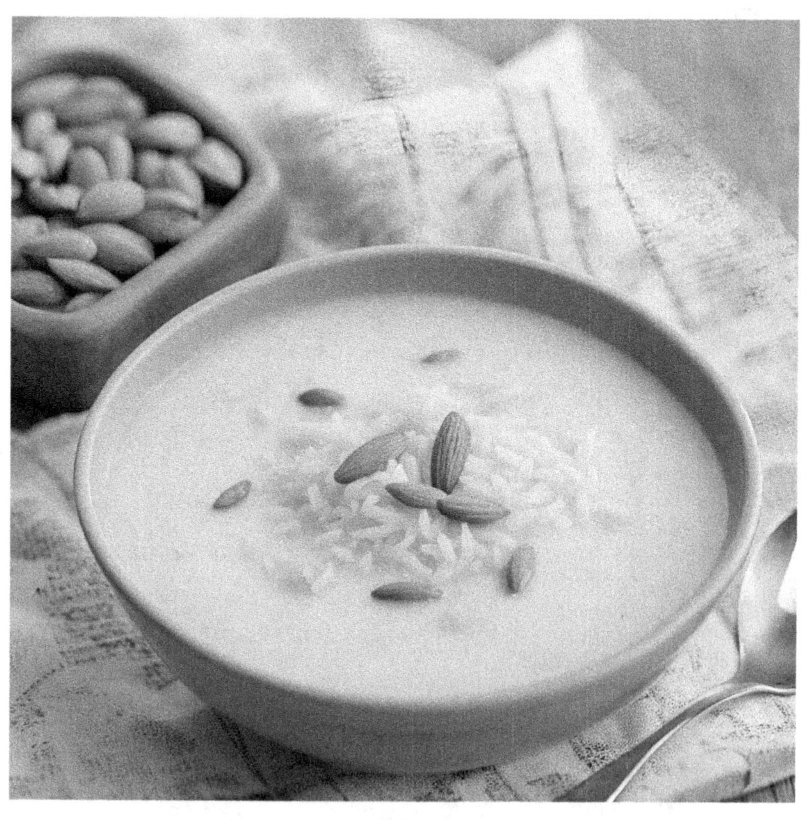

14. Parsnip Soup
Ingredients:
- 2 lbs parsnips, peeled and chopped
- 4 cups vegetable broth
- 1 onion, chopped
- 1 tbsp olive oil
- 1 tsp ground ginger

Instructions:
1. In a large pot, heat olive oil over medium heat. Sauté onion until translucent.
2. Add parsnips and vegetable broth. Bring to a boil, then simmer for 30 minutes until parsnips are tender.
3. Puree the soup until smooth, then reheat and stir in ground ginger.

Nutrition Info Per Serving:
- Calories: 210
- Protein: 2g
- Carbohydrates: 49g
- Fat: 4g

Serves: 4
Cooking Time: 40 minutes

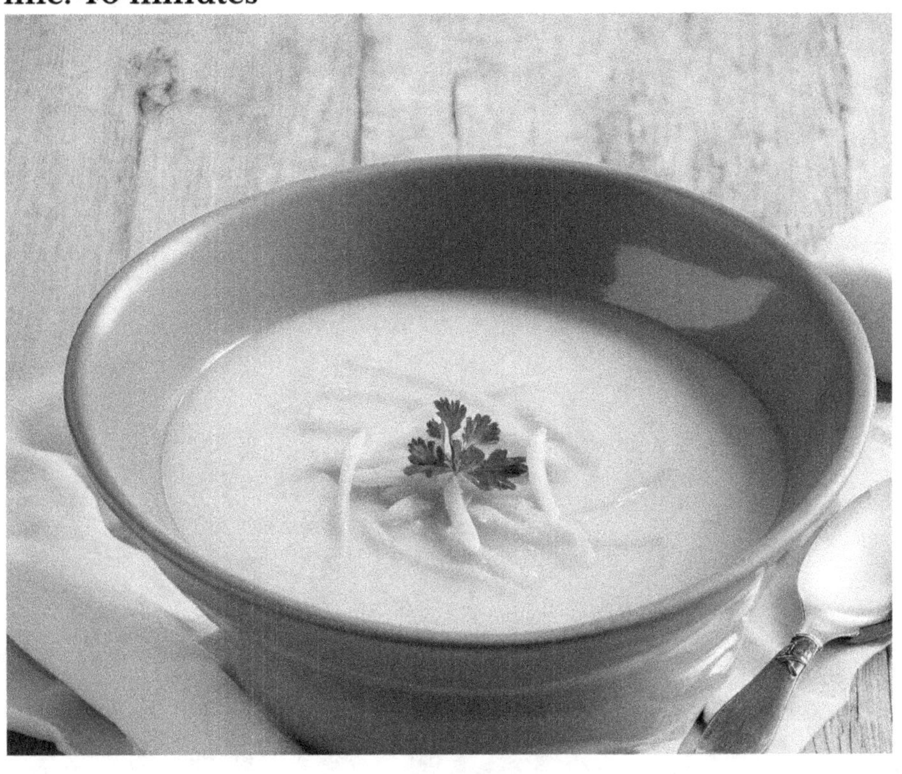

15. Zucchini Ribbon Salad

Ingredients:

- 2 zucchinis, cut into thin ribbons with a peeler
- 1/4 cup chopped walnuts
- 1/4 cup feta cheese, crumbled
- 2 tbsp olive oil
- 1 tbsp balsamic vinegar

Instructions:

1. In a large bowl, combine zucchini ribbons, walnuts, and feta cheese.
2. Drizzle with olive oil and balsamic vinegar, then toss gently to combine.

Nutrition Info Per Serving:

- Calories: 200
- Protein: 5g
- Carbohydrates: 8g
- Fat: 17g

Serves: 4

Cooking Time: 10 minutes

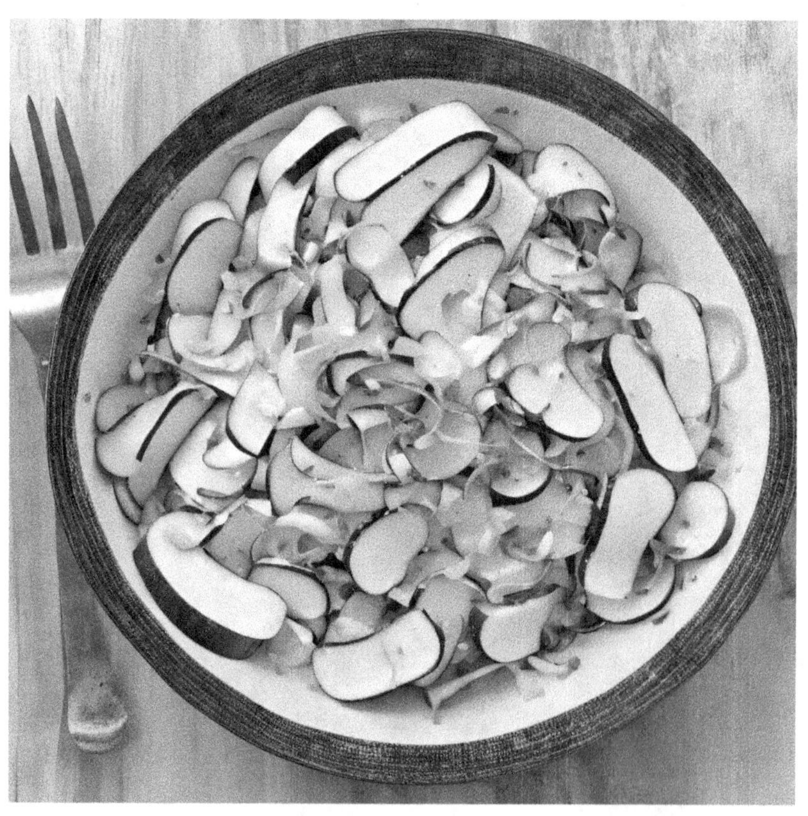

16. Simple Mixed Greens Salad

Ingredients:

- 4 cups mixed salad greens
- 1/4 cup sliced almonds
- 2 tbsp olive oil
- 1 tbsp balsamic vinegar

Instructions:

1. In a large salad bowl, toss mixed greens and sliced almonds.
2. Drizzle with olive oil and balsamic vinegar, then toss again to coat.

Nutrition Info Per Serving:

- Calories: 150
- Protein: 3g
- Carbohydrates: 6g
- Fat: 13g

Serves: 4

Cooking Time: 5 minutes

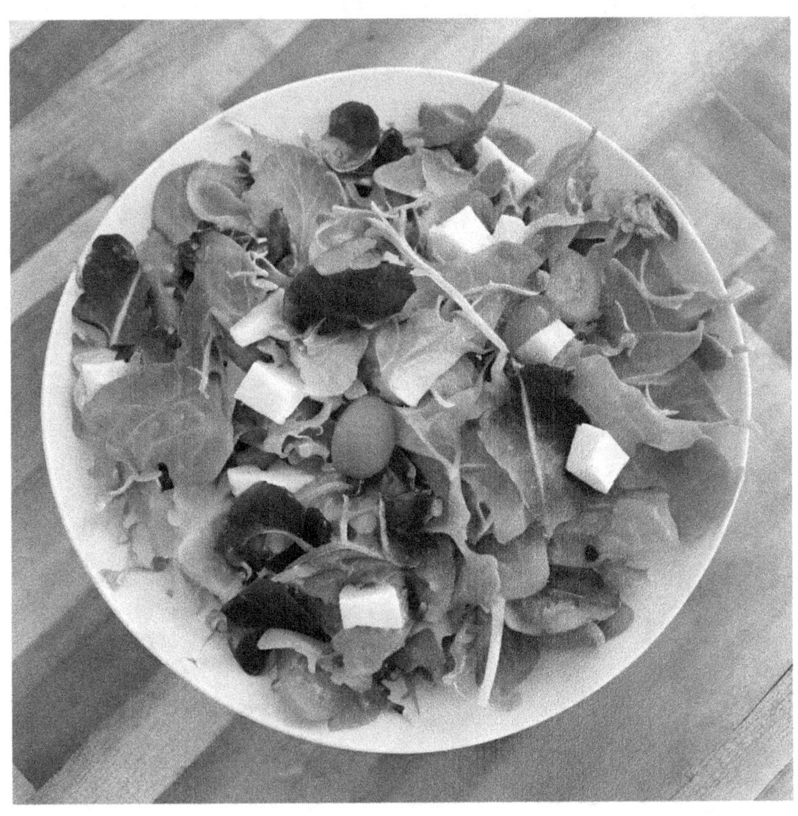

17. Roasted Bell Pepper Salad

Ingredients:

- 4 bell peppers, assorted colors, roasted and sliced
- 1/4 cup pine nuts
- 2 tbsp olive oil
- 1 tbsp balsamic vinegar

Instructions:

1. In a salad bowl, combine roasted bell peppers and pine nuts.
2. Drizzle with olive oil and balsamic vinegar, then toss to combine.

Nutrition Info Per Serving:

- Calories: 200
- Protein: 2g
- Carbohydrates: 12g
- Fat: 16g

Serves: 4

Cooking Time: 15 minutes (excluding roasting time)

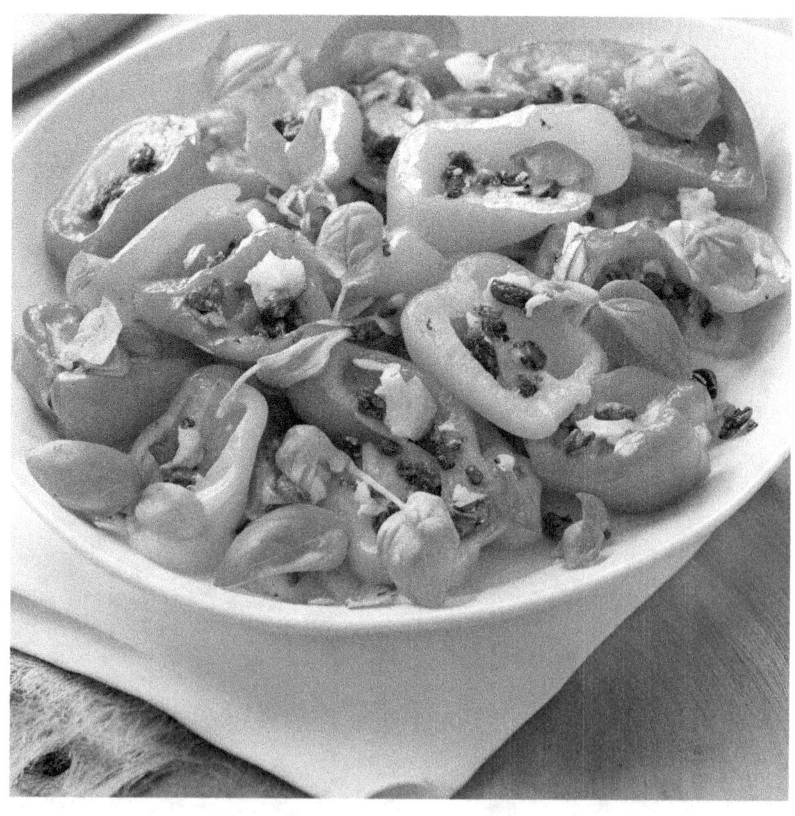

18. Rice Salad with Peas

Ingredients:

- 2 cups cooked rice (preferably cold)
- 1 cup green peas, cooked and cooled
- 1/2 cup chopped red bell pepper
- 1/4 cup chopped fresh parsley
- 2 tbsp olive oil
- 1 tbsp white vinegar

Instructions:

1. In a large bowl, combine cooked rice, green peas, red bell pepper, and parsley.
2. Drizzle with olive oil and white vinegar, then toss well to mix all ingredients evenly.

Nutrition Info Per Serving:

- Calories: 230
- Protein: 5g
- Carbohydrates: 38g
- Fat: 7g

Serves: 4
Cooking Time: 10 minutes

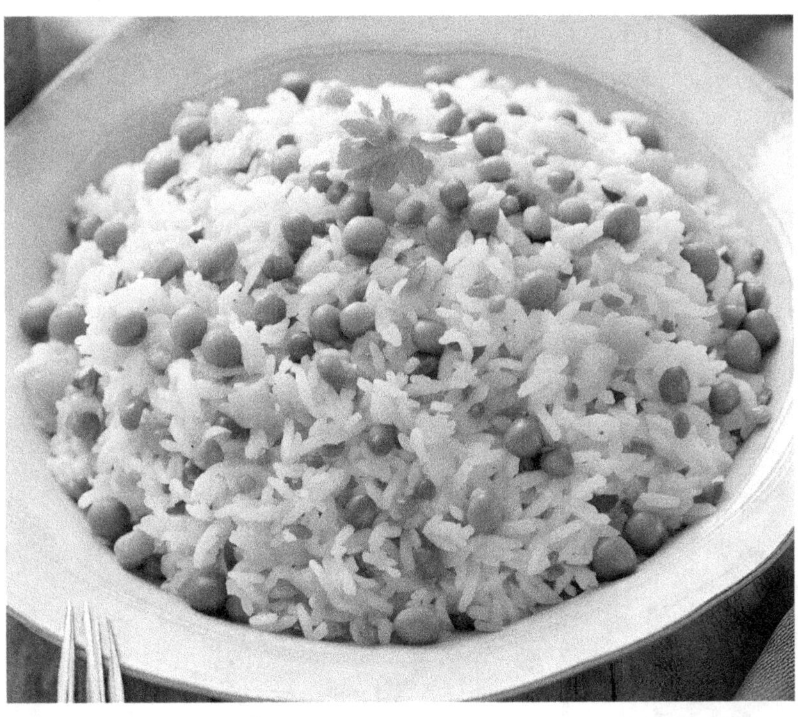

19. Quinoa and Cucumber Salad

Ingredients:

- 1 cup quinoa, cooked and cooled
- 1 cucumber, diced
- 1/4 cup chopped mint
- 1/4 cup feta cheese, crumbled
- 2 tbsp olive oil
- 1 tbsp lemon juice (optional for those who can tolerate it)

Instructions:

1. In a large salad bowl, combine quinoa, cucumber, mint, and feta cheese.
2. Drizzle with olive oil and lemon juice (if using), then toss gently to combine.

Nutrition Info Per Serving:

- Calories: 220
- Protein: 8g
- Carbohydrates: 30g
- Fat: 8g

Serves: 4

Cooking Time: 10 minutes

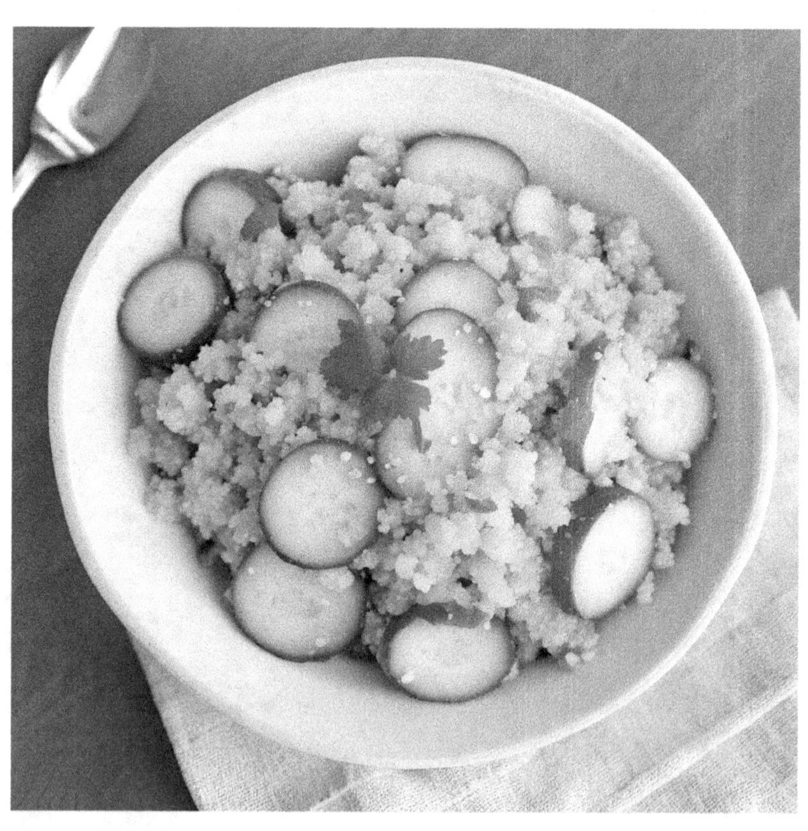

20. Potato Salad
Ingredients:

- 3 large potatoes, boiled, peeled, and cubed
- 1/2 cup plain yogurt
- 1/4 cup chopped green onions
- 1/4 cup chopped fresh dill
- 2 tbsp olive oil

Instructions:

1. In a large bowl, combine cubed potatoes, yogurt, green onions, and dill.
2. Drizzle with olive oil and gently mix until all ingredients are well combined.

Nutrition Info Per Serving:

- Calories: 260
- Protein: 6g
- Carbohydrates: 38g
- Fat: 10g

Serves: 4
Cooking Time: 30 minutes (includes time for boiling potatoes)

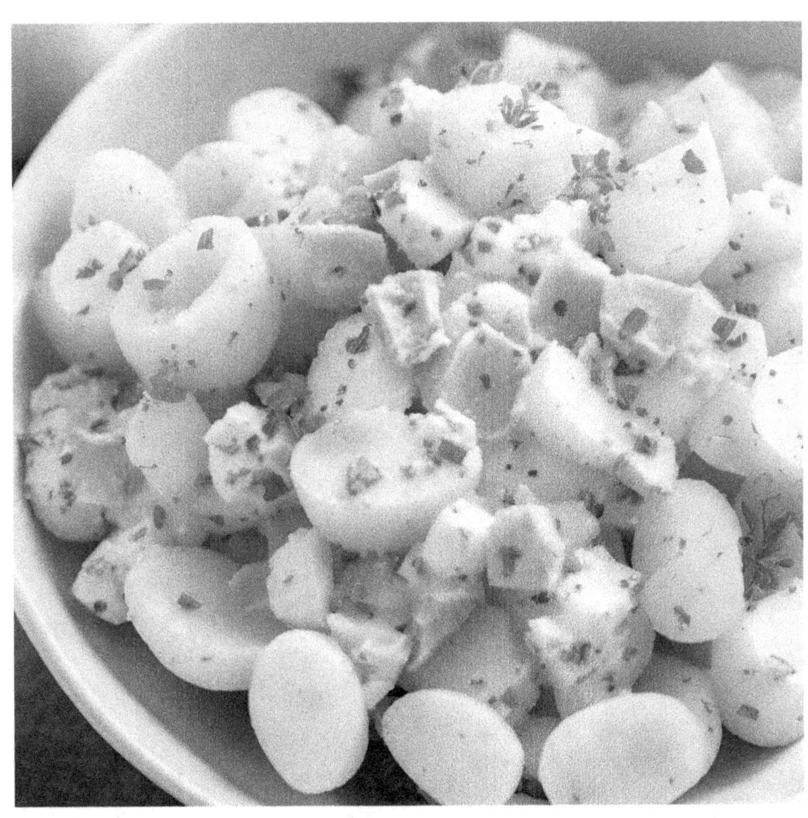

21. Pear and Spinach Salad

Ingredients:

- 4 cups fresh spinach
- 2 pears, cored and sliced
- 1/4 cup walnuts, chopped
- 1/4 cup blue cheese, crumbled
- 2 tbsp olive oil
- 1 tbsp balsamic vinegar

Instructions:

1. In a large salad bowl, combine spinach, sliced pears, walnuts, and blue cheese.
2. Drizzle with olive oil and balsamic vinegar, then toss gently to combine all the ingredients.

Nutrition Info Per Serving:

- Calories: 220
- Protein: 5g
- Carbohydrates: 20g
- Fat: 14g

Serves: 4

Cooking Time: 10 minutes

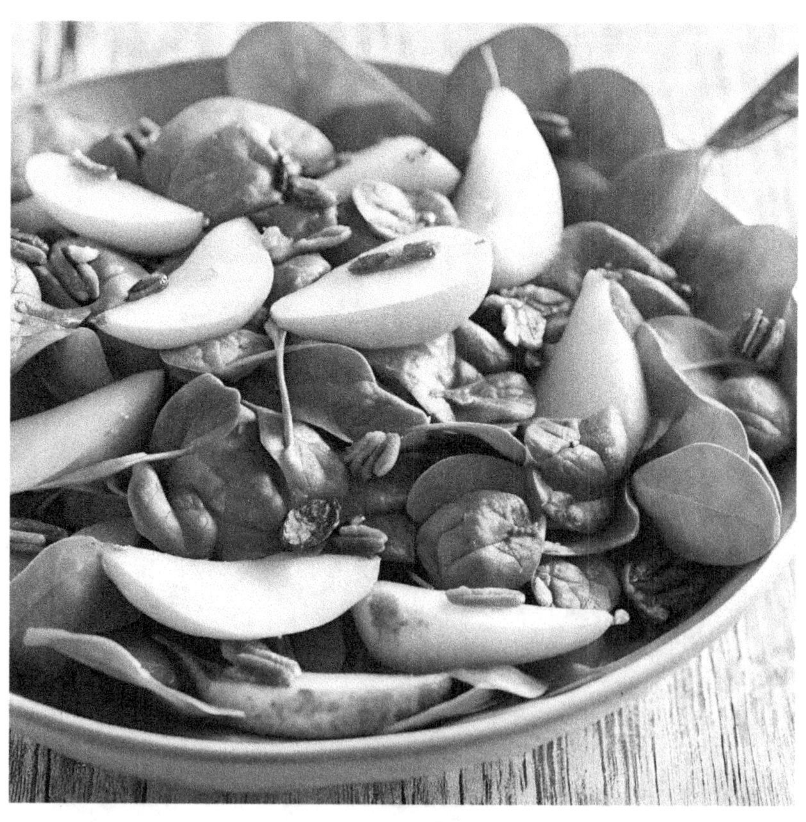

Snacks & Sides Recipes

1. Baked Pear Chips
Ingredients:
- 3 ripe pears
- 1 tsp cinnamon

Instructions:
1. Preheat the oven to 225°F (110°C).
2. Core the pears and slice them very thinly.
3. Arrange pear slices in a single layer on a baking sheet lined with parchment paper.
4. Sprinkle with cinnamon.
5. Bake for 1.5 to 2 hours, turning halfway through, until the pear slices are dried and crisp.
6. Allow to cool before serving.

Nutrition Info Per Serving:
- Calories: 50
- Protein: 0g
- Carbohydrates: 13g
- Fat: 0g

Serves: 4
Cooking Time: 2 hours

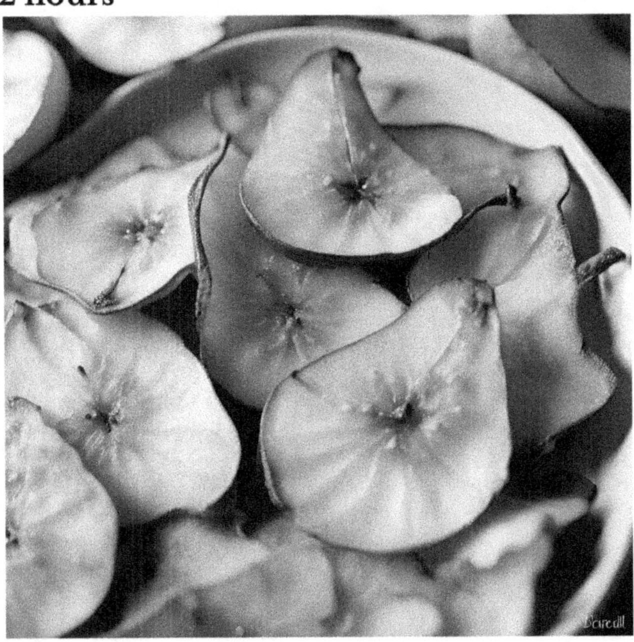

2. Oatmeal Cookies

Ingredients:

- 1 cup rolled oats
- 1/2 cup almond flour
- 1/4 cup honey or maple syrup
- 1 egg
- 1/2 cup unsweetened applesauce
- 1 tsp vanilla extract
- 1/2 tsp cinnamon

Instructions:

1. Preheat the oven to 350°F (175°C).
2. In a large bowl, mix together oats, almond flour, and cinnamon.
3. In another bowl, whisk together honey, egg, applesauce, and vanilla extract.
4. Combine the wet and dry ingredients until well mixed.
5. Drop spoonfuls of the mixture onto a baking sheet lined with parchment paper.
6. Bake for 10-12 minutes until the edges are golden brown.
7. Allow to cool on the baking sheet before transferring to a wire rack.

Nutrition Info Per Serving:

- Calories: 100
- Protein: 3g
- Carbohydrates: 15g
- Fat: 4g

Serves: 12 cookies

Cooking Time: 12 minutes

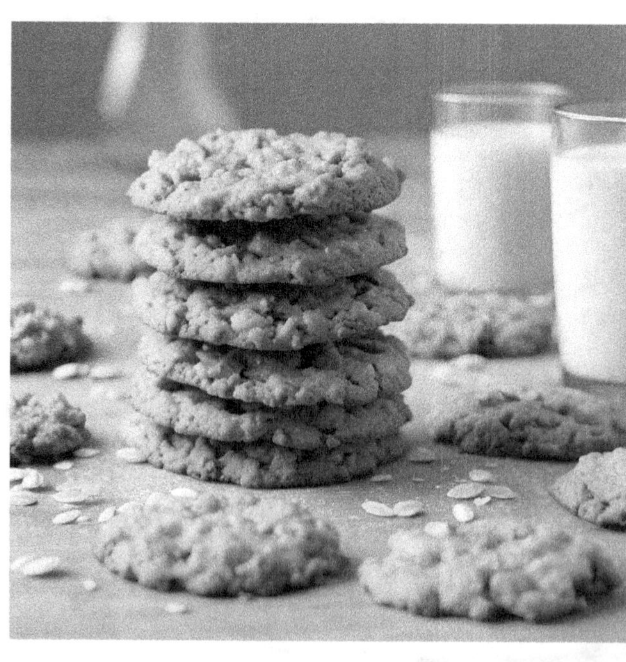

3. Rice Cakes with Almond Butter

Ingredients:

- 4 rice cakes
- 4 tbsp almond butter
- Optional toppings: sliced bananas or a drizzle of honey

Instructions:

1. Spread 1 tablespoon of almond butter evenly over each rice cake.
2. If desired, top each with sliced banana or a drizzle of honey for extra sweetness.

Nutrition Info Per Serving (without optional toppings):

- Calories: 150
- Protein: 4g
- Carbohydrates: 18g
- Fat: 8g

Serves: 4
Cooking Time: 5 minutes

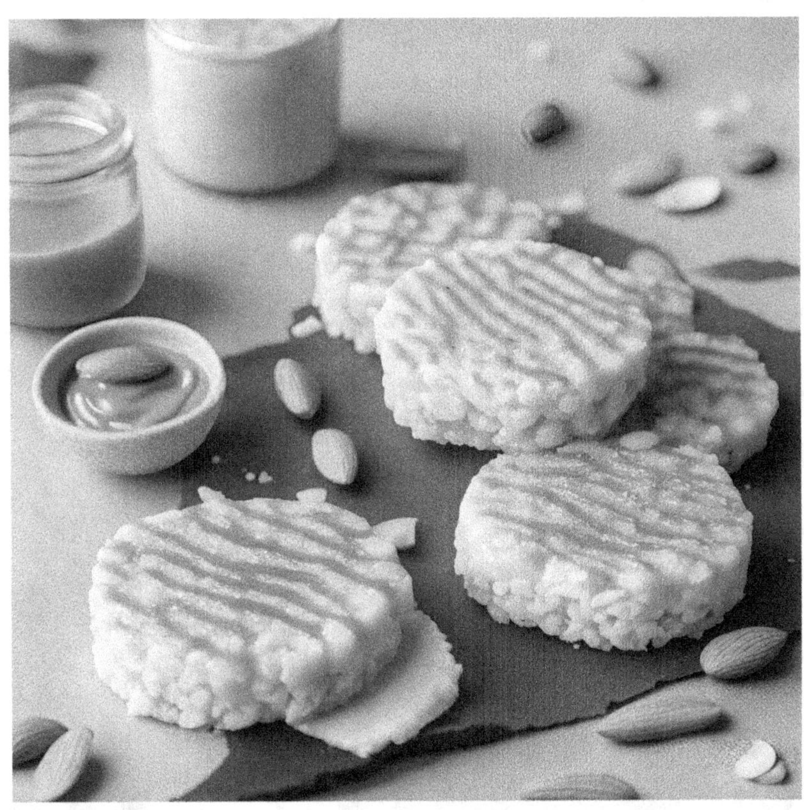

4. Roasted Almonds

Ingredients:

- 2 cups raw almonds
- 1 tbsp olive oil
- 1 tsp dried rosemary

Instructions:

1. Preheat the oven to 350°F (175°C).
2. In a bowl, toss almonds with olive oil and dried rosemary until well coated.
3. Spread the almonds in a single layer on a baking sheet.
4. Roast in the oven for 10-12 minutes, stirring occasionally, until golden and fragrant.
5. Allow to cool before serving.

Nutrition Info Per Serving:

- Calories: 170
- Protein: 6g
- Carbohydrates: 6g
- Fat: 15g

Serves: 8

Cooking Time: 12 minutes

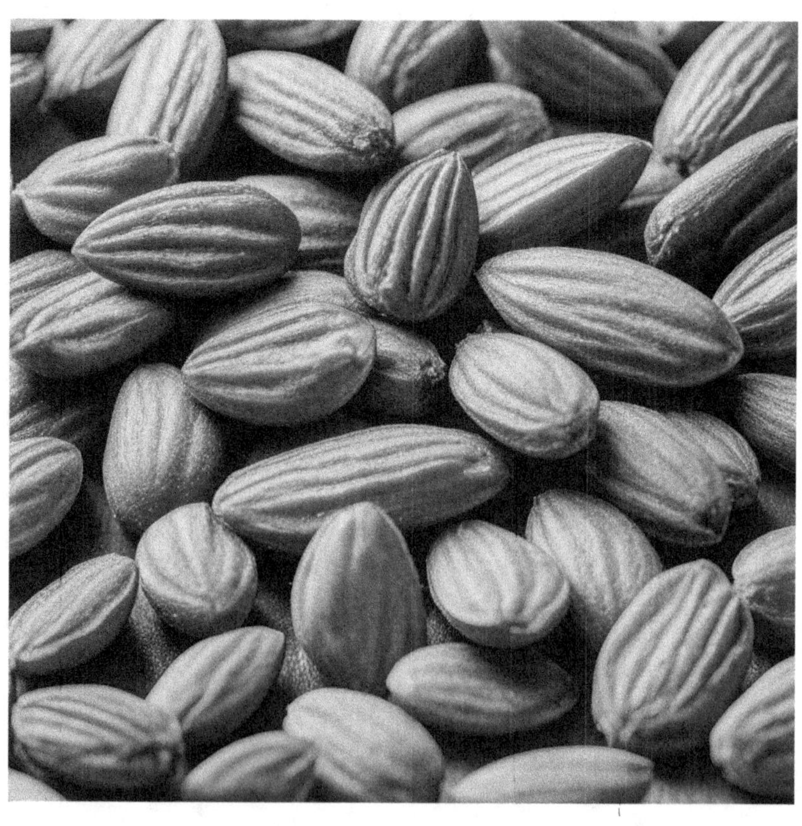

5. Baked Sweet Potato Fries

Ingredients:

- 2 large sweet potatoes, peeled and sliced into fries
- 2 tbsp olive oil
- 1 tsp paprika

Instructions:

1. Preheat the oven to 425°F (220°C).
2. Toss sweet potato fries with olive oil and paprika in a bowl until evenly coated.
3. Spread the fries in a single layer on a baking sheet.
4. Bake for 20-25 minutes, turning once halfway through, until crispy and golden.
5. Serve warm.

Nutrition Info Per Serving:

- Calories: 140
- Protein: 2g
- Carbohydrates: 24g
- Fat: 4g

Serves: 4
Cooking Time: 25 minutes

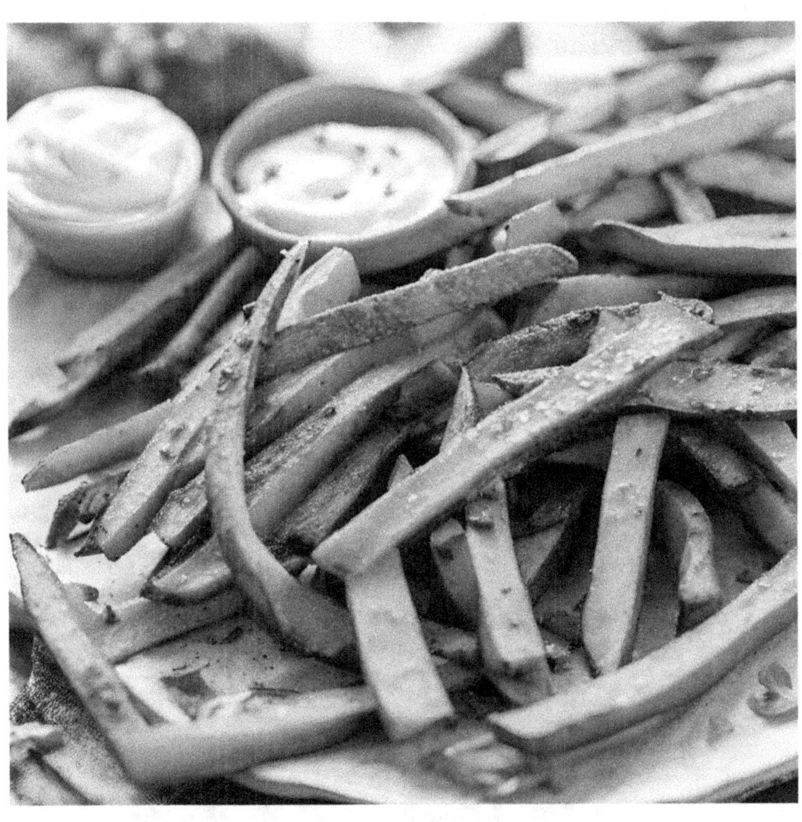

6. Zucchini Muffins

Ingredients:

- 2 cups grated zucchini
- 1 cup almond flour
- 1/2 cup oat flour
- 1/4 cup olive oil
- 1/4 cup honey
- 2 eggs
- 1 tsp vanilla extract
- 1 tsp cinnamon

Instructions:

1. Preheat the oven to 375°F (190°C).
2. In a large bowl, mix together grated zucchini, almond flour, oat flour, and cinnamon.
3. In another bowl, whisk together eggs, olive oil, honey, and vanilla extract.
4. Combine the wet and dry ingredients until well mixed.
5. Spoon the batter into a greased muffin tin.
6. Bake for 20-25 minutes until a toothpick inserted into the center of a muffin comes out clean.
7. Allow to cool before serving.

Nutrition Info Per Serving:

- Calories: 200
- Protein: 6g
- Carbohydrates: 18g
- Fat: 12g

Serves: 12 muffins

Cooking Time: 25 minutes

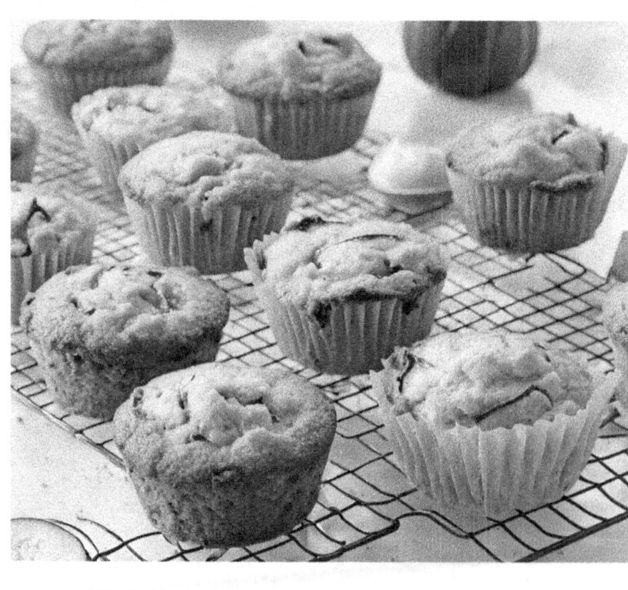

7. Melon Balls

Ingredients:

- 1 cantaloupe
- 1 honeydew melon

Instructions:

1. Using a melon baller, scoop out balls from both the cantaloupe and honeydew melon.
2. Mix the melon balls in a serving bowl and chill in the refrigerator before serving.

Nutrition Info Per Serving:

- Calories: 50
- Protein: 1g
- Carbohydrates: 12g
- Fat: 0g

Serves: 6
Cooking Time: 10 minutes (plus chilling time)

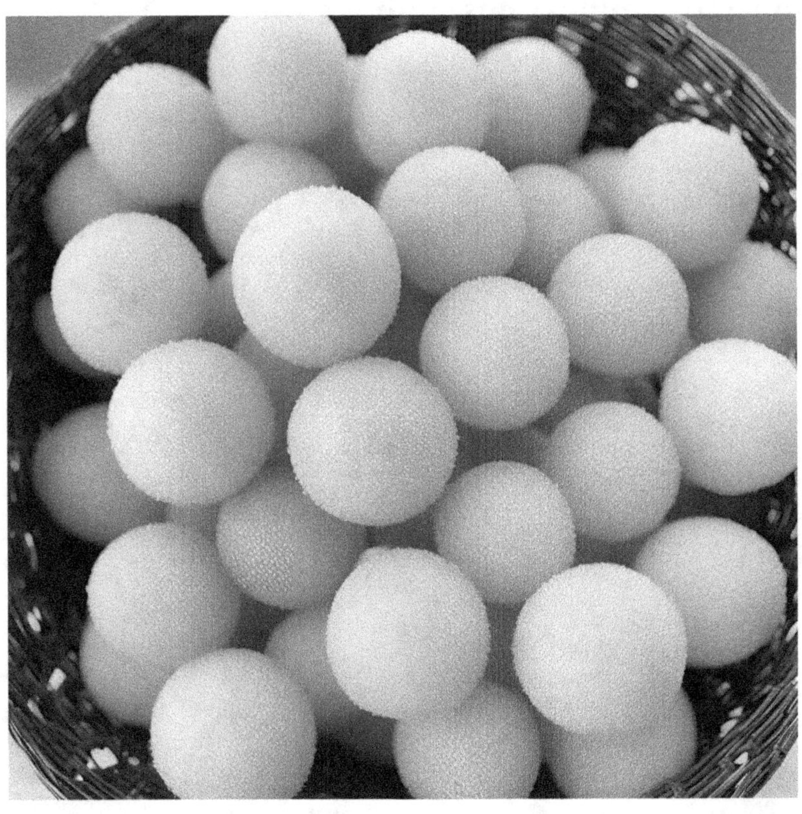

8. Puffed Rice Bars

Ingredients:

- 3 cups puffed rice
- 1/2 cup honey
- 1/2 cup peanut butter

Instructions:

1. In a saucepan, heat honey and peanut butter over low heat until smooth and well combined.
2. Remove from heat and stir in puffed rice until evenly coated.
3. Press the mixture into a greased 9x9 inch baking pan.
4. Chill in the refrigerator for 1 hour, or until set.
5. Cut into bars and serve.

Nutrition Info Per Serving:

- Calories: 150
- Protein: 4g
- Carbohydrates: 22g
- Fat: 6g

Serves: 12 bars

Cooking Time: 10 minutes (plus chilling time)

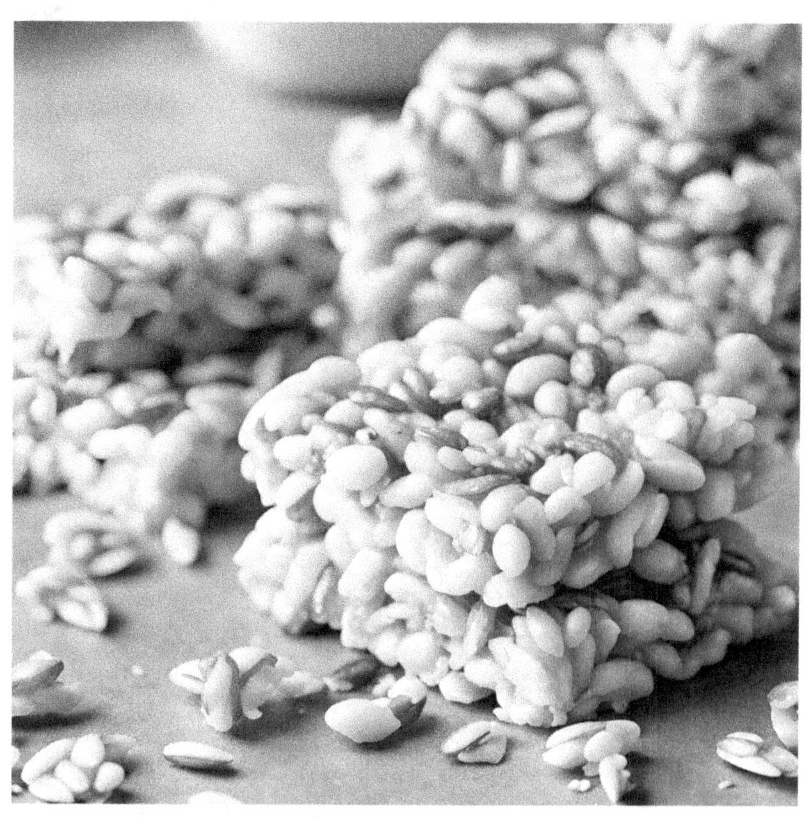

9. Banana Bread

Ingredients:

- 3 ripe bananas, mashed
- 2 cups oat flour
- 1/4 cup olive oil
- 1/4 cup honey
- 2 eggs
- 1 tsp vanilla extract
- 1 tsp baking soda

Instructions:

1. Preheat the oven to 350°F (175°C).
2. In a large bowl, combine mashed bananas, oat flour, and baking soda.
3. In another bowl, whisk together eggs, olive oil, honey, and vanilla extract.
4. Mix the wet ingredients into the dry ingredients until well combined.
5. Pour the batter into a greased loaf pan.
6. Bake for 50-55 minutes, or until a toothpick inserted into the center comes out clean.
7. Allow to cool before slicing.

Nutrition Info Per Serving:

- Calories: 200
- Protein: 4g
- Carbohydrates: 32g
- Fat: 7g

Serves: 10
Cooking Time: 55 minutes

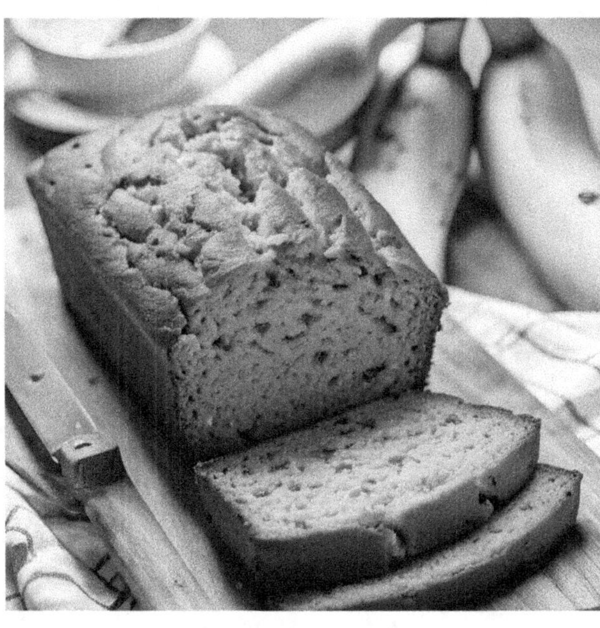

10. Mashed Potatoes

Ingredients:

- 4 large potatoes, peeled and cubed
- 1/4 cup cream
- 2 tbsp butter
- 1 tsp dried parsley

Instructions:

1. Boil the potato cubes in water until tender, about 20 minutes.
2. Drain the potatoes and return them to the pot.
3. Add cream and butter, and mash until smooth and creamy.
4. Stir in dried parsley and serve warm.

Nutrition Info Per Serving:

- Calories: 250
- Protein: 4g
- Carbohydrates: 38g
- Fat: 10g

Serves: 4

Cooking Time: 30 minutes

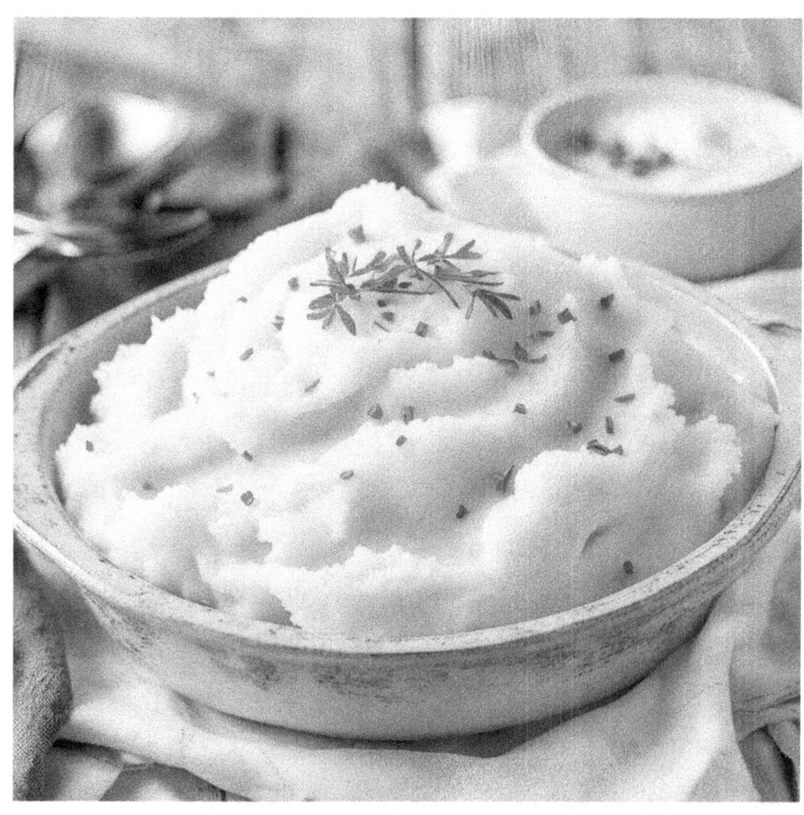

11. Steamed Asparagus

Ingredients:

- 1 lb asparagus, trimmed
- 1 tbsp olive oil
- 1 tsp lemon zest (optional, for those who can tolerate it)

Instructions:

1. Bring water to a boil in a pot fitted with a steamer basket.
2. Place asparagus in the basket, cover, and steam for about 3-5 minutes until tender but still crisp.
3. Drizzle with olive oil and sprinkle with lemon zest if using.

Nutrition Info Per Serving:

- Calories: 60
- Protein: 3g
- Carbohydrates: 4g
- Fat: 4g

Serves: 4

Cooking Time: 5 minutes

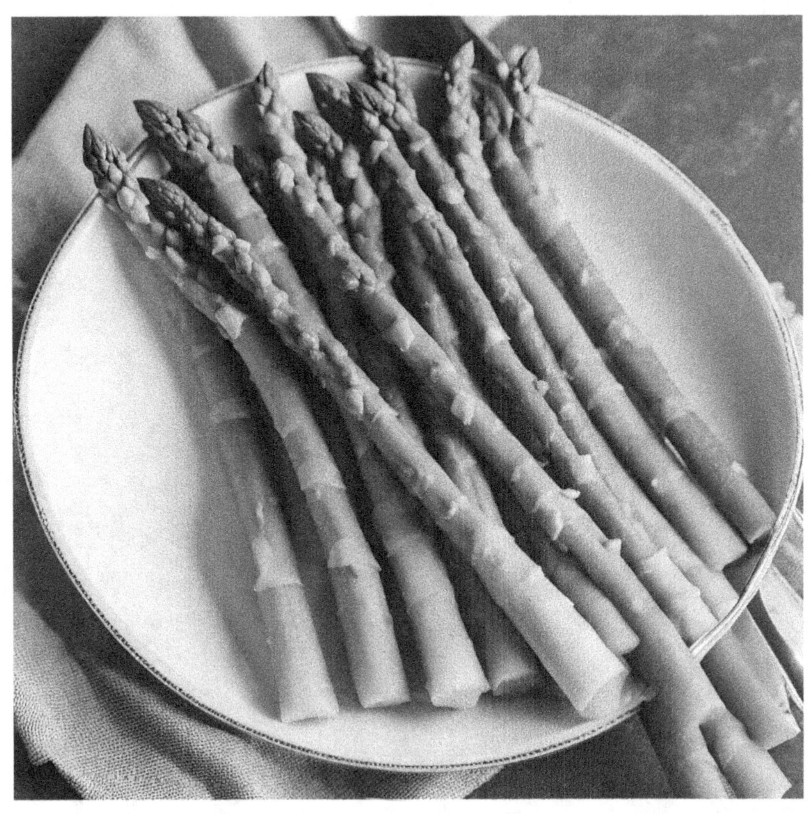

12. Herbed Quinoa

Ingredients:
- 1 cup quinoa
- 2 cups water
- 1 tbsp olive oil
- 1/4 cup chopped fresh herbs (such as parsley and thyme)

Instructions:
1. Rinse quinoa under cold water until water runs clear.
2. In a saucepan, combine quinoa, water, and olive oil. Bring to a boil.
3. Reduce heat to low, cover, and simmer for 15 minutes or until water is absorbed.
4. Stir in fresh herbs before serving.

Nutrition Info Per Serving:
- Calories: 210
- Protein: 8g
- Carbohydrates: 30g
- Fat: 6g

Serves: 4
Cooking Time: 20 minutes

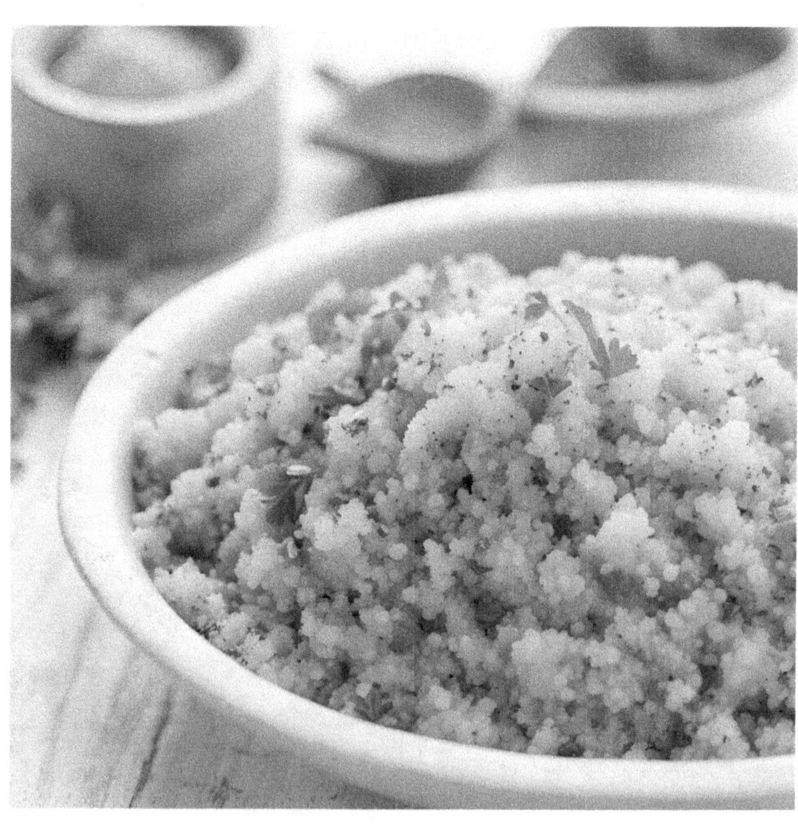

13. Garlic-Free Coleslaw

Ingredients:

- 4 cups shredded cabbage
- 1 cup shredded carrots
- 1/2 cup mayonnaise
- 1 tbsp apple cider vinegar
- 1 tbsp sugar

Instructions:

1. In a large bowl, combine cabbage and carrots.
2. In a separate bowl, whisk together mayonnaise, apple cider vinegar, and sugar.
3. Pour the dressing over the cabbage mixture and toss to coat evenly.

Nutrition Info Per Serving:

- Calories: 180
- Protein: 1g
- Carbohydrates: 12g
- Fat: 14g

Serves: 4

Cooking Time: 10 minutes

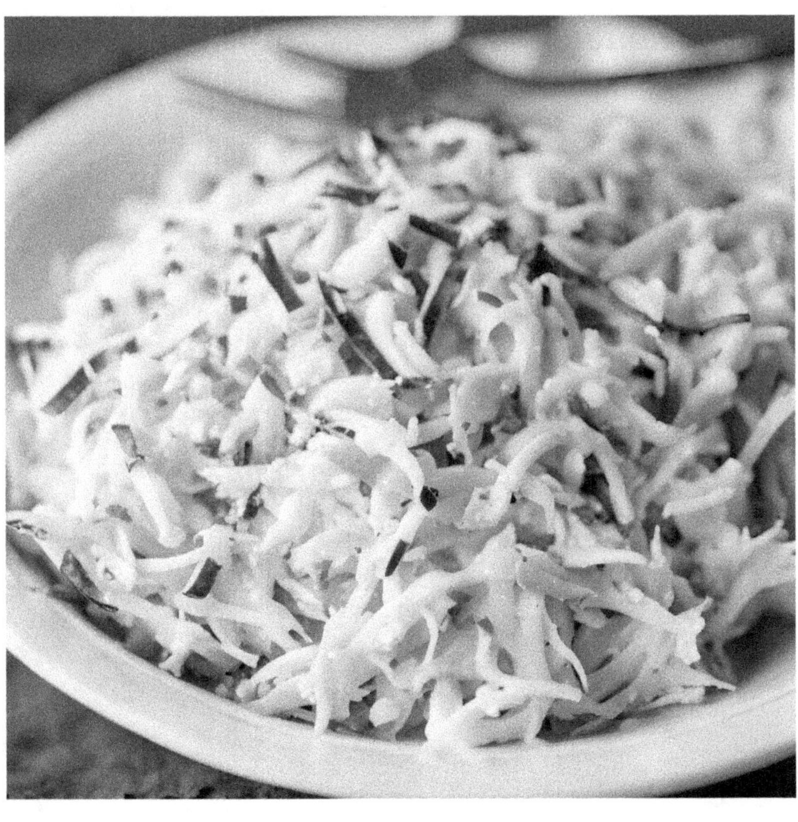

14. Plain Risotto

Ingredients:

- 1 cup Arborio rice
- 4 cups chicken or vegetable broth
- 1 onion, finely chopped
- 1 tbsp olive oil
- 1/4 cup grated Parmesan cheese

Instructions:

1. In a large saucepan, heat olive oil over medium heat. Add onion and cook until translucent.
2. Add rice and stir to coat with oil for about 2 minutes.
3. Add broth 1/2 cup at a time, stirring constantly, until each addition is absorbed before adding the next.
4. Once rice is creamy and al dente, stir in Parmesan cheese.

Nutrition Info Per Serving:

- Calories: 260
- Protein: 6g
- Carbohydrates: 45g
- Fat: 6g

Serves: 4

Cooking Time: 30 minutes

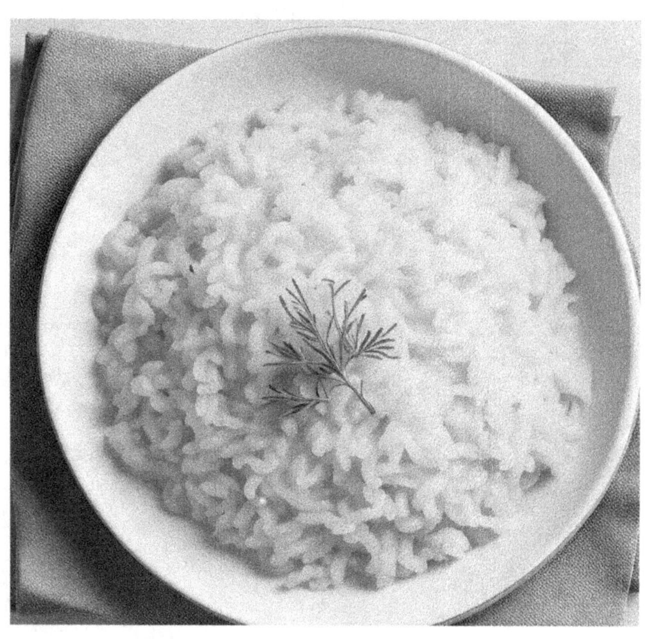

15. Baked Polenta

Ingredients:

- 1 cup polenta (cornmeal)
- 4 cups water
- 1 tbsp olive oil
- 1/4 cup grated Parmesan cheese

Instructions:

1. Preheat oven to 350°F (175°C).
2. Bring water to a boil and gradually whisk in polenta.
3. Reduce heat and simmer, stirring frequently, until thickened.
4. Stir in olive oil and half of the Parmesan cheese.
5. Pour polenta into a greased baking dish, sprinkle with remaining cheese.
6. Bake for 20-25 minutes until golden and set.

Nutrition Info Per Serving:

- Calories: 220
- Protein: 5g
- Carbohydrates: 31g
- Fat: 8g

Serves: 4
Cooking Time: 45 minutes

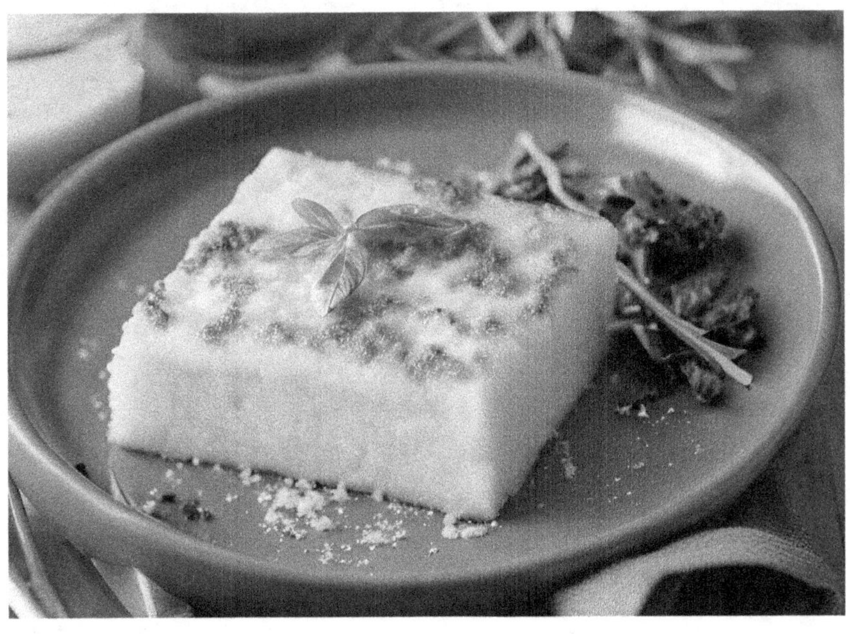

16. Butternut Squash Cubes

Ingredients:

- 1 large butternut squash, peeled and cubed
- 2 tbsp olive oil
- 1 tsp cinnamon

Instructions:

1. Preheat oven to 400°F (200°C).
2. Toss butternut squash cubes with olive oil and cinnamon.
3. Spread on a baking sheet and roast for 25-30 minutes until tender.

Nutrition Info Per Serving:

- Calories: 140
- Protein: 2g
- Carbohydrates: 20g
- Fat: 7g

Serves: 4
Cooking Time: 30 minutes

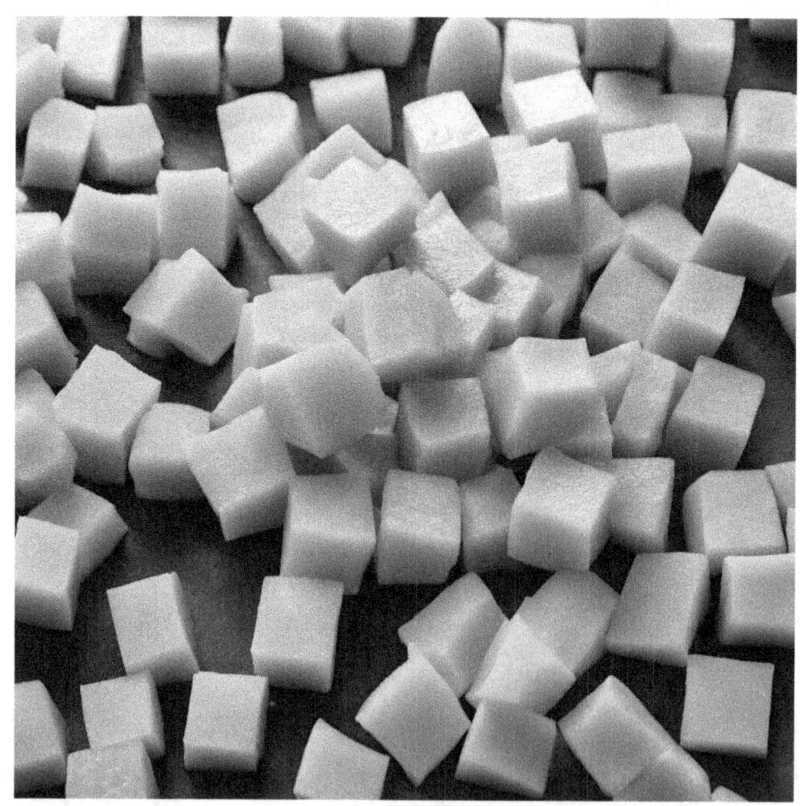

17. Green Pea Mash
Ingredients:
- 2 cups green peas, cooked
- 1 tbsp olive oil
- 1/4 cup mint leaves, chopped (optional)

Instructions:
1. In a bowl, mash the cooked peas with a potato masher or fork.
2. Stir in olive oil and mint leaves if using.
3. Serve warm or at room temperature.

Nutrition Info Per Serving:
- Calories: 120
- Protein: 5g
- Carbohydrates: 16g
- Fat: 4.5g

Serves: 4
Cooking Time: 10 minutes (excluding cooking peas)

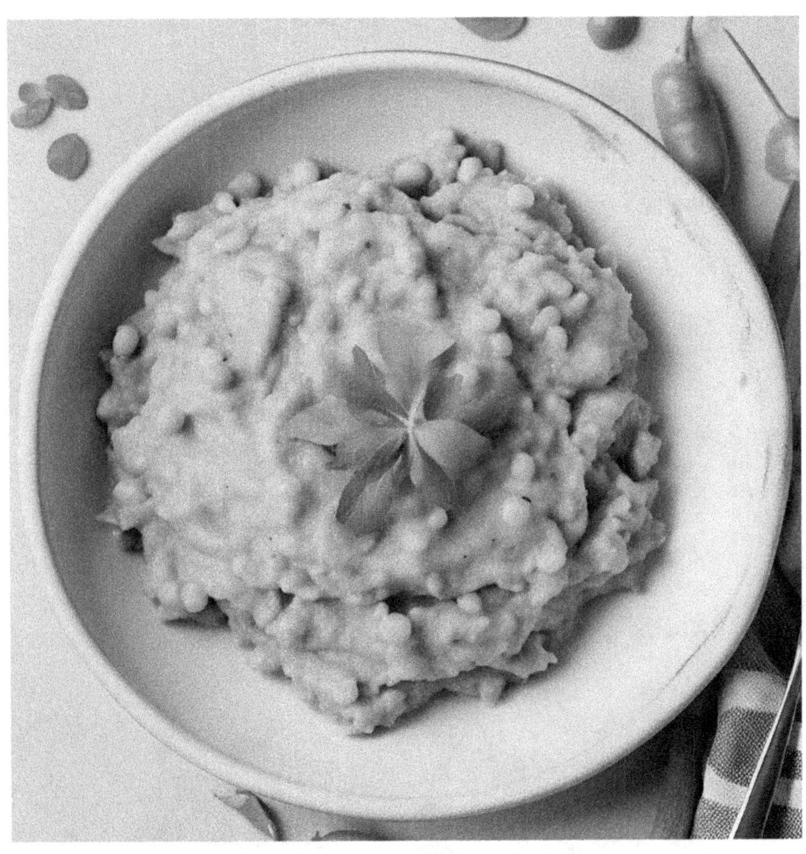

18. Plain Naan Bread

Ingredients:

- 2 cups all-purpose flour
- 1/2 tsp sugar
- 1/2 tsp baking powder
- 1/2 cup milk
- 1/4 cup plain yogurt
- 1 tbsp olive oil

Instructions:

1. In a large bowl, combine flour, sugar, and baking powder.
2. In another bowl, mix milk, yogurt, and olive oil.
3. Gradually add the wet ingredients to the dry, mixing to form a soft dough.
4. Knead on a floured surface until smooth.
5. Divide dough into balls and roll out into thin discs.
6. Cook each disc in a hot skillet until bubbles form, then flip and cook until golden on the other side.

Nutrition Info Per Serving:

- Calories: 180
- Protein: 5g
- Carbohydrates: 30g
- Fat: 4g

Serves: 8

Cooking Time: 15 minutes

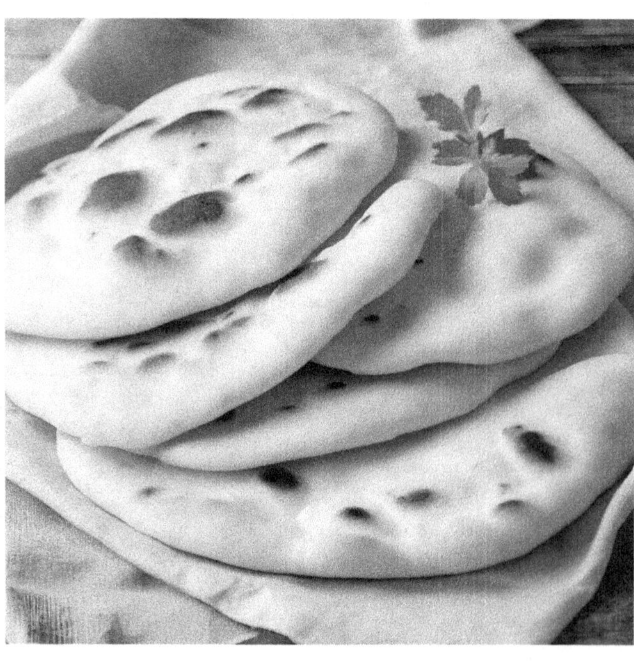

19. Fennel Salad

Ingredients:

- 2 fennel bulbs, thinly sliced
- 1/4 cup sliced almonds
- 2 tbsp olive oil
- 1 tbsp balsamic vinegar

Instructions:

1. In a salad bowl, combine thinly sliced fennel and sliced almonds.
2. Drizzle with olive oil and balsamic vinegar, then toss to coat evenly.

Nutrition Info Per Serving:

- Calories: 130
- Protein: 2g
- Carbohydrates: 10g
- Fat: 10g

Serves: 4
Cooking Time: 10 minutes

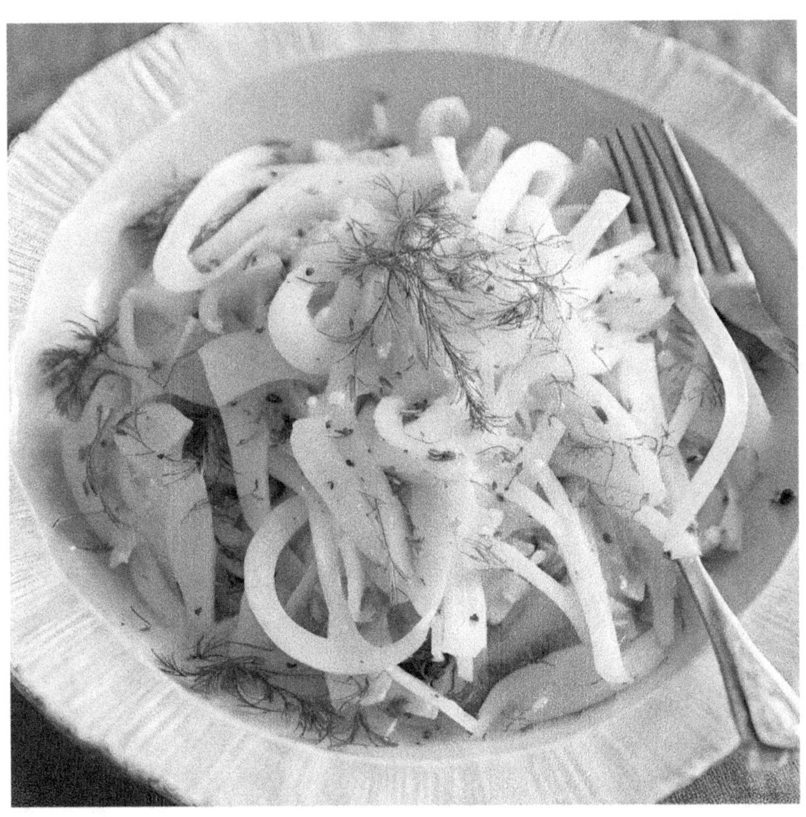

20. Herb-Seasoned Broccoli

Ingredients:

- 1 lb broccoli florets
- 2 tbsp olive oil
- 1 tsp dried herbs (such as thyme and rosemary)

Instructions:

1. Preheat oven to 400°F (200°C).
2. Toss broccoli florets with olive oil and dried herbs.
3. Spread on a baking sheet and roast for 20 minutes until crisp and tender.

Nutrition Info Per Serving:

- Calories: 120
- Protein: 4g
- Carbohydrates: 10g
- Fat: 8g

Serves: 4

Cooking Time: 20 minutes

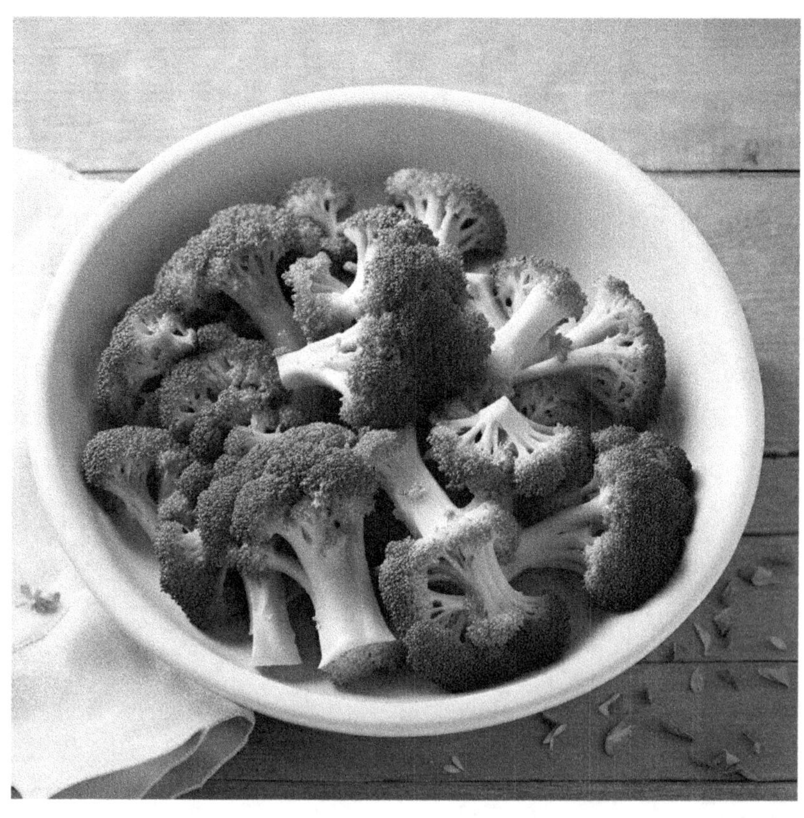

Week 1

Day 1:
- **Breakfast:** Pear Oatmeal
- **Lunch:** Chicken Salad
- **Dinner:** Herb-Roasted Turkey Breast
- **Snack:** Baked Pear Chips

Day 2:
- **Breakfast:** Blueberry Smoothie
- **Lunch:** Vegetable and Barley Soup
- **Dinner:** Maple Glazed Salmon
- **Snack:** Rice Cakes with Almond Butter

Day 3:
- **Breakfast:** Banana Pancakes
- **Lunch:** Turkey Sandwich
- **Dinner:** Beef Sirloin with Parsley
- **Snack:** Oatmeal Cookies

Day 4:
- **Breakfast:** Apple Cinnamon Porridge
- **Lunch:** Cucumber and Dill Salad
- **Dinner:** Chicken Alfredo Pasta
- **Snack:** Puffed Rice Bars

Day 5:
- **Breakfast:** Rice Pudding
- **Lunch:** Roasted Chicken Breast
- **Dinner:** Roasted Duck with Wild Rice
- **Snack:** Banana Bread

Day 6:
- **Breakfast:** Pumpkin Oatmeal
- **Lunch:** Pasta with Olive Oil and Garlic
- **Dinner:** Rabbit Stew with Vegetables
- **Snack:** Roasted Almonds

Day 7:
- **Breakfast:** Avocado Rice Cakes
- **Lunch:** Beef Stew
- **Dinner:** Grilled Lamb Chops with Mint
- **Snack:** Melon Balls

Week 2

Day 8:
- **Breakfast:** Sweet Potato Hash
- **Lunch:** Quinoa Salad
- **Dinner:** Garlic Butter Baked Cod
- **Snack:** Baked Sweet Potato Fries

Day 9:
- **Breakfast:** Zucchini Bread
- **Lunch:** Baked Potato with Chives
- **Dinner:** Pasta Primavera
- **Snack:** Zucchini Muffins

Day 10:
- **Breakfast:** Quinoa Breakfast Bowl
- **Lunch:** Spinach and Cheese Quesadilla
- **Dinner:** Roasted Turkey and Sweet Potato
- **Snack:** Mashed Potatoes

Day 11:
- **Breakfast:** Buckwheat Pancakes
- **Lunch:** Mild White Fish Tacos
- **Dinner:** Creamy Polenta with Mushrooms
- **Snack:** Butternut Squash Cubes

Day 12:
- **Breakfast:** Omelette with Fresh Herbs
- **Lunch:** Chicken and Rice Soup
- **Dinner:** Herb-Roasted Quail
- **Snack:** Green Pea Mash

Day 13:
- **Breakfast:** Pumpkin Smoothie
- **Lunch:** Chicken and Avocado Salad
- **Dinner:** Baked Polenta
- **Snack:** Plain Naan Bread

Day 14:
- **Breakfast:** Baked Oatmeal
- **Lunch:** Carrot and Raisin Salad
- **Dinner:** Venison Stew
- **Snack:** Fennel Salad

Week 3

Day 15:
- **Breakfast:** Barley Porridge
- **Lunch:** Green Bean Soup
- **Dinner:** Mushroom Risotto
- **Snack:** Herb-Seasoned Broccoli

Day 16:
- **Breakfast:** Savory Vegetable Pancakes
- **Lunch:** Leek and Potato Soup
- **Dinner:** Flounder with Parsley Sauce
- **Snack:** Plain Risotto

Day 17:
- **Breakfast:** Vanilla Almond Milk Porridge
- **Lunch:** Apple Walnut Salad
- **Dinner:** Steamed Asparagus
- **Snack:** Rice Salad with Peas

Day 18:
- **Breakfast:** Rice and Almond Soup
- **Lunch:** Pear and Spinach Salad
- **Dinner:** Herbed Quinoa
- **Snack:** Simple Mixed Greens Salad

Day 19:
- **Breakfast:** Parsnip Soup
- **Lunch:** Quinoa and Cucumber Salad
- **Dinner:** Chicken Noodle Soup
- **Snack:** Potato Salad

Day 20:
- **Breakfast:** Oatmeal Soup
- **Lunch:** Roasted Bell Pepper Salad
- **Dinner:** Plain Risotto
- **Snack:** Garlic-Free Coleslaw

Day 21:
- **Breakfast:** Corn Chowder
- **Lunch:** Zucchini Ribbon Salad
- **Dinner:** Egg Drop Soup
- **Snack:** Steamed Asparagus

Week 4

Day 22:
- **Breakfast:** Pear Oatmeal
- **Lunch:** Broccoli Cheese Soup
- **Dinner:** Lemon-Free Chicken Piccata
- **Snack:** Puffed Rice Bars

Day 23:
- **Breakfast:** Rice Pudding
- **Lunch:** Turkey Sandwich
- **Dinner:** Grilled Cheese Sandwich
- **Snack:** Baked Pear Chips

Day 24:
- **Breakfast:** Banana Pancakes
- **Lunch:** Cucumber and Dill Salad
- **Dinner:** Pasta with Peas and Ham
- **Snack:** Rice Cakes with Almond Butter

Day 25:
- **Breakfast:** Apple Cinnamon Porridge
- **Lunch:** Roasted Chicken Breast
- **Dinner:** Baked Potato with Chives
- **Snack:** Oatmeal Cookies

Day 26:
- **Breakfast:** Pumpkin Oatmeal
- **Lunch:** Pasta with Olive Oil and Garlic
- **Dinner:** Chicken Noodle Soup
- **Snack:** Banana Bread

Day 27:
- **Breakfast:** Avocado Rice Cakes
- **Lunch:** Beef Stew
- **Dinner:** Beef Sirloin with Parsley
- **Snack:** Roasted Almonds

Day 28:
- **Breakfast:** Sweet Potato Hash
- **Lunch:** Quinoa Salad
- **Dinner:** Herbed Baked Pollock
- **Snack:** Melon Balls

Week 5

Day 29:
- **Breakfast:** Buckwheat Pancakes
- **Lunch:** Chicken and Avocado Salad
- **Dinner:** Roasted Duck with Wild Rice
- **Snack:** Baked Sweet Potato Fries

Day 30:
- **Breakfast:** Omelette with Fresh Herbs
- **Lunch:** Chicken and Rice Soup
- **Dinner:** Maple Glazed Salmon
- **Snack:** Zucchini Muffins

Day 31:
- **Breakfast:** Pumpkin Smoothie
- **Lunch:** Spinach and Cheese Quesadilla
- **Dinner:** Herb-Roasted Turkey Breast
- **Snack:** Mashed Potatoes

Day 32:
- **Breakfast:** Baked Oatmeal
- **Lunch:** Beef Sirloin with Parsley
- **Dinner:** Garlic Butter Baked Cod
- **Snack:** Butternut Squash Cubes

Day 33:
- **Breakfast:** Quinoa Breakfast Bowl
- **Lunch:** Baked Potato with Chives
- **Dinner:** Pasta Primavera
- **Snack:** Green Pea Mash

Day 34:
- **Breakfast:** Barley Porridge
- **Lunch:** Mild White Fish Tacos
- **Dinner:** Grilled Lamb Chops with Mint
- **Snack:** Plain Naan Bread

Day 35:
- **Breakfast:** Savory Vegetable Pancakes
- **Lunch:** Carrot and Raisin Salad
- **Dinner:** Venison Stew
- **Snack:** Fennel Salad

Week 6

Day 36:

- **Breakfast:** Vanilla Almond Milk Porridge
- **Lunch:** Green Bean Soup
- **Dinner:** Mushroom Risotto
- **Snack:** Herb-Seasoned Broccoli

Day 37:

- **Breakfast:** Oatmeal Soup
- **Lunch:** Leek and Potato Soup
- **Dinner:** Flounder with Parsley Sauce
- **Snack:** Plain Risotto

Day 38:

- **Breakfast:** Rice and Almond Soup
- **Lunch:** Pear and Spinach Salad
- **Dinner:** Herbed Quinoa
- **Snack:** Simple Mixed Greens Salad

Day 39:

- **Breakfast:** Parsnip Soup
- **Lunch:** Quinoa and Cucumber Salad
- **Dinner:** Chicken Noodle Soup
- **Snack:** Potato Salad

Day 40:

- **Breakfast:** Corn Chowder
- **Lunch:** Zucchini Ribbon Salad
- **Dinner:** Egg Drop Soup
- **Snack:** Steamed Asparagus

Day 41:

- **Breakfast:** Asparagus Cream Soup
- **Lunch:** Rice Salad with Peas
- **Dinner:** Steamed Asparagus
- **Snack:** Baked Polenta

Day 42:

- **Breakfast:** Barley and Mushroom Soup
- **Lunch:** Roasted Bell Pepper Salad
- **Dinner:** Plain Risotto
- **Snack:** Garlic-Free Coleslaw

Week 7

Day 43:
- **Breakfast:** Herb-Roasted Turkey Breast
- **Lunch:** Broccoli Cheese Soup
- **Dinner:** Lemon-Free Chicken Piccata
- **Snack:** Puffed Rice Bars

Day 44:
- **Breakfast:** Rice Pudding
- **Lunch:** Turkey Sandwich
- **Dinner:** Grilled Cheese Sandwich
- **Snack:** Baked Pear Chips

Day 45:
- **Breakfast:** Banana Pancakes
- **Lunch:** Cucumber and Dill Salad
- **Dinner:** Pasta with Peas and Ham
- **Snack:** Rice Cakes with Almond Butter

Day 46:
- **Breakfast:** Apple Cinnamon Porridge
- **Lunch:** Roasted Chicken Breast
- **Dinner:** Baked Potato with Chives
- **Snack:** Oatmeal Cookies

Day 47:
- **Breakfast:** Pumpkin Oatmeal
- **Lunch:** Pasta with Olive Oil and Garlic
- **Dinner:** Chicken Noodle Soup
- **Snack:** Banana Bread

Day 48:
- **Breakfast:** Avocado Rice Cakes
- **Lunch:** Beef Stew
- **Dinner:** Beef Sirloin with Parsley
- **Snack:** Roasted Almonds

Day 49:
- **Breakfast:** Sweet Potato Hash
- **Lunch:** Quinoa Salad
- **Dinner:** Herbed Baked Pollock
- **Snack:** Melon Balls

Week 8

Day 50:
- **Breakfast:** Buckwheat Pancakes
- **Lunch:** Chicken and Avocado Salad
- **Dinner:** Roasted Duck with Wild Rice
- **Snack:** Baked Sweet Potato Fries

Day 51:
- **Breakfast:** Omelette with Fresh Herbs
- **Lunch:** Chicken and Rice Soup
- **Dinner:** Maple Glazed Salmon
- **Snack:** Zucchini Muffins

Day 52:
- **Breakfast:** Pumpkin Smoothie
- **Lunch:** Spinach and Cheese Quesadilla
- **Dinner:** Herb-Roasted Turkey Breast
- **Snack:** Mashed Potatoes

Day 53:
- **Breakfast:** Baked Oatmeal
- **Lunch:** Beef Sirloin with Parsley
- **Dinner:** Garlic Butter Baked Cod
- **Snack:** Butternut Squash Cubes

Day 54:
- **Breakfast:** Quinoa Breakfast Bowl
- **Lunch:** Baked Potato with Chives
- **Dinner:** Pasta Primavera
- **Snack:** Green Pea Mash

Day 55:
- **Breakfast:** Barley Porridge
- **Lunch:** Mild White Fish Tacos
- **Dinner:** Grilled Lamb Chops with Mint
- **Snack:** Plain Naan Bread

Day 56:
- **Breakfast:** Savory Vegetable Pancakes
- **Lunch:** Carrot and Raisin Salad
- **Dinner:** Venison Stew
- **Snack:** Fennel Salad

MEAL PLANNER JOURNAL

	BREAKFAST	LUNCH	DINNER	SNACKS
MON				
TUE				
WED				
THU				
FRI				
SAT				
SUN				

What are your main symptoms of interstitial cystitis, and how do they affect your daily life?

MEAL PLANNER JOURNAL

	BREAKFAST	LUNCH	DINNER	SNACKS
MON				
TUE				
WED				
THU				
FRI				
SAT				
SUN				

List three goals you hope to achieve by following the interstitial cystitis diet.

MEAL PLANNER JOURNAL

	BREAKFAST	LUNCH	DINNER	SNACKS
MON				
TUE				
WED				
THU				
FRI				
SAT				
SUN				

What foods do you currently eat that you suspect might trigger your IC symptoms?

MEAL PLANNER JOURNAL

	BREAKFAST	LUNCH	DINNER	SNACKS
MON				
TUE				
WED				
THU				
FRI				
SAT				
SUN				

How do you feel about making dietary changes to manage your IC symptoms?

MEAL PLANNER JOURNAL

	BREAKFAST	LUNCH	DINNER	SNACKS
MON				
TUE				
WED				
THU				
FRI				
SAT				
SUN				

Describe a typical day's meals and snacks before starting the IC diet.

MEAL PLANNER JOURNAL

	BREAKFAST	LUNCH	DINNER	SNACKS
MON				
TUE				
WED				
THU				
FRI				
SAT				
SUN				

What are your biggest concerns or challenges when it comes to following the IC diet?

MEAL PLANNER JOURNAL

	BREAKFAST	LUNCH	DINNER	SNACKS
MON				
TUE				
WED				
THU				
FRI				
SAT				
SUN				

Identify three bladder-friendly foods you are excited to incorporate into your diet.

MEAL PLANNER JOURNAL

	BREAKFAST	LUNCH	DINNER	SNACKS
MON				
TUE				
WED				
THU				
FRI				
SAT				
SUN				

How do you plan to handle dining out or social events while following the IC diet?

MEAL PLANNER JOURNAL

	BREAKFAST	LUNCH	DINNER	SNACKS
MON				
TUE				
WED				
THU				
FRI				
SAT				
SUN				

What new recipes or cooking techniques are you interested in trying on the IC diet?

MEAL PLANNER JOURNAL

	BREAKFAST	LUNCH	DINNER	SNACKS
MON				
TUE				
WED				
THU				
FRI				
SAT				
SUN				

Describe any previous attempts you've made to manage your IC symptoms through diet. What worked and what didn't?

MEAL PLANNER JOURNAL

	BREAKFAST	LUNCH	DINNER	SNACKS
MON				
TUE				
WED				
THU				
FRI				
SAT				
SUN				

How will you stay motivated to stick to the IC diet during difficult times?

MEAL PLANNER JOURNAL

	BREAKFAST	LUNCH	DINNER	SNACKS
MON				
TUE				
WED				
THU				
FRI				
SAT				
SUN				

Reflect on how you expect your quality of life to improve by following the IC diet.

Scan the QR code below to get a surprise bonus!